AGING AGGRESSIVELY:

How to Avoid the US Health-Care Crisis

THOMAS JONES, MD,
AND JOHN COTTON, MS

BETSY M. CHALFIN, M.ED., EDITOR

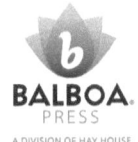

BALBOA.
PRESS

A DIVISION OF HAY HOUSE

Balboa Press books may be ordered through booksellers or by contacting:

Balboa Press
A Division of Hay House
1663 Liberty Drive
Bloomington, IN 47403
www.balboapress.com
1 (877) 407-4847

Because of the dynamic nature of the Internet, any web addresses or
links contained in this book may have changed since publication and
may no longer be valid. The views expressed in this work are solely those
of the author and do not necessarily reflect the views of the publisher,
and the publisher hereby disclaims any responsibility for them.

The author of this book does not dispense medical advice or prescribe the use
of any technique as a form of treatment for physical, emotional, or medical
problems without the advice of a physician, either directly or indirectly. The
intent of the author is only to offer information of a general nature to help you
in your quest for emotional and spiritual well-being. In the event you use any
of the information in this book for yourself, which is your constitutional right,
the author and the publisher assume no responsibility for your actions.

Any people depicted in stock imagery provided by Thinkstock are models,
and such images are being used for illustrative purposes only.
Certain stock imagery © Thinkstock.

Printed in the United States of America.

ISBN: 978-1-4525-8660-1 (sc)
ISBN: 978-1-4525-8662-5 (hc)
ISBN: 978-1-4525-8661-8 (e)

Library of Congress Control Number: 2013920067

Balboa Press rev. date: 11/11/2013

Contents

1. Take Charge of Your Health 1
2. A Social Perspective 7

What We Need to Do As Individuals

3. Frequent Minor Problems of Elders 19
4. Maintaining an Active and Fulfilling Lifestyle 23
5. Obtaining Appropriate Physical and Mental Support,
   Health Advice and Nursing Care 29
6. Educating Your Physician About Quality of Life Care 42
7. When Medications, Diagnostic Tests and Procedures
   Are Needed and When They Are Not 54

Issues Regarding Public Policy of Health Care

8. The Politics of Your Health Care 59
9. Examples of Health Care Insurance Plans and
   Government Health Care Taxation Approaches 68
10. Medicare and Medicaid Health Plans—Designed to Fail? 84
11. Recent Proposals to Reform Medicare 93

Personal Things to Remember

12. The Importance of Humor, Domestic Pets, Music and
    Interpersonal Relationships 107
13. Memories are an important part of aging—Both the
    Good and the Bad 115

Conclusion

14. Aging is A Wonderful Process But It Must Be Done
    Aggressively 123

Afterword 125

Appendices

Appendix A. Confusing Language is a Major Problem in
             Understanding Medication for Young and Old 129
Appendix B. A Conceptual Societal Health
             Program for Elders 135

References 147

About the Authors 151

1

Take Charge of Your Health

This book is about growing older, about taking charge of your health, about understanding present health care policies, and about feeling secure and enjoying the process. It is also a clarion call to those of us who are older adults to take advantage of two important facts: we are a significant numerical force in society, and we can and should be certain that our voices are heard in every aspect of social and medical planning. This book was stimulated by, and is a follow up of, the book "Taking Charge of Your Health" by John Burton and William Hall. That book sets the stage, we hope this one fills in some of the details.

The book is divided into three sections. The first (chapters 1–7) describes what we face each day of our aging lives and what we can do to interact with our health care providers in a positive but assertive way. The second (chapters 8–11 and the appendices) is a primer on current health care policy in the United States and internationally, so that we can better understand decisions politicians and physicians are making thus enabling us to make relevant contributions to the process. The third (chapters 12 and 13) offers nuts and bolts suggestions and some personal insight about maintaining a sense of humor, achieving self-fulfillment, and reflecting on our memories while facing the important issues of health, medical care, and end-of-life decisions.

Thomas C. Jones has been a highly respected research physician trained in infectious diseases, international medicine, and public health. He is emeritus professor of medicine at Weill-Cornell School of Medicine, where he did his own internship and residency, and later was one of the most popular professors of parasitology and infectious diseases. He has cared for patients in private practice, on hospital wards, in an army hospital in the Philippines during the Vietnam War, and in the refugee camps of Thailand and along the Pakistan-Afghanistan border. He has published over 200 scientific articles, chapters in the most important medical textbooks, and his own book titled *Medical Care of Refugees* (Oxford University Press, 1986). He was the first editor of the *Brazilian Journal of Infectious Diseases*—the first English-language medical journal ever published in South America. His research on toxoplasmosis provided ground-breaking insight into that disease process, and his collaboration with physicians and researchers in Brazil and Haiti brought him international respect among his peers and created a rich environment for study for the medical students, residents, and researchers who worked abroad with funding from his grants. Dr. Jones is in a unique position to address the issues of our faltering health care system and recommend a solution—specifically, what we can do to obtain the care we need and head off a potential health crisis, for our own lives and for our society. Now that he is retired from professional medicine and outside of the mainstream, Dr. Jones's somewhat irreverent view is precisely what makes his opinions relevant today.

As contributing author, John F. Cotton has contributed two chapters (2 and 11) and Appendix B to this book. His views are pertinent based on his many years of experience in state government, originating and administering the details of health care-related federal programs and policies. In addition, his views on how those programs affect quality of life for elders and our real social obligations make his contribution especially valuable.

The editor, Betsy Chalfin, adds another dimension based on her years as a copyeditor for Thomas C. Jones at Cornell University Medical College and at the *Brazilian Journal of Infectious Diseases*, and from her years of experience as a program coordinator in international refugee relief and as a hospital administrator.

There are a number of familiar quotations that suggest how we should think about aging and we have selected two in particular to set the tone for this book. Dylan Thomas wrote, "Do not go gentle into that good night . . ." The second is a quote from the character Old Lodge Skins in the movie *Little Big Man* based on the book by Thomas Berger. Old Lodge Skins thought it was his time to go to the Happy Hunting Ground so he climbed up into the mountains and waited for Nature to take its course. After waiting awhile, he realized he was still alive and concluded, "Sometimes the magic just does not work!"

Our primary focus here is health care for elders—what is wrong with it and what we can do to make it suit our needs. You will learn that health care is not just about medicine but it is also a complex mix of social attitudes and personal and political will.

There are many examples of special and often discriminatory treatment of elders in our society—like forced retirement regardless of productivity; periodic medical reports required to engage in active sports despite the fact that they are in good health; exclusion from certain social events that are planned for a younger population; or participation in a musical group or chorus that prefers a more youthful public relations image. There is often a lot of fun and peace of mind associated with getting older, but for the situations that fail to meet our needs or expectations, we advocate an aggressive approach to challenge and change them.

When one considers the issue of health care and what can be done to improve it, especially the care directed specifically toward the aging population, we find a number of powerful influences in play. We find that lawyers enthusiastic about generating class-action legal challenges for their own financial gain, regulatory agencies influenced by numerous lobbyists anxious to direct the purchasing power of elders, and politicians elected or removed by the increasingly elder demographic are the powerful sources of potential change of the system—not physicians.

As participants in the health care bureaucracy, the authors learned that physicians alone are unable or unwilling to define the life-enhancing support systems needed for their patients and translate them into appropriate delivery of health care. Ever increasing pressures on health care providers makes this so. These pressures include administrative guidelines and insurance reimbursement requirements that impose time limits allotted for a physician to spend with each patient even though the physician believes more time is necessary for adequate evaluation and care; constant advertising that suggests nearly miraculous effects of a specific prescription medication that misleads patients and prompts them to question their physician's recommendations; and finally, intellectual and financial rewards that drive young physicians toward medical specialization rather than general medicine—each of these pressure tactics work against a physician's need and desire to focus on the overall health status and life quality needs of his or her patient.

There are a number of hidden features affecting the social welfare of elders that must be explored. The plethora of medications prescribed for the aging population is a vivid example. In their book, Burton and Hill quoted the famous physician, writer, and social critic Oliver Wendell Holmes. To paraphrase that quote, ". . . almost all medications prescribed to patients would do better to be thrown into the sea—a good move for humanity although probably not so good for the fish." The multitude of prescribed medications are supposed to allow a patient to reach old age but the clinical studies, the statistical analyses of these studies, and information on how they apply to special sub-groups are often not available. So, a 75-year-old patient is instructed to take a certain medication to improve his or her chance of survival even though the drug studies were done on specific at-risk groups between 30 and 60 years old. The logical question here is, "Why not focus a study on those over age 70 whom the drug is usually prescribed for?" The answer is almost always that the subgroup analysis of the targeted population would alter the power of the statistical result—in other words, the pharmaceutical companies could not exaggerate the beneficial power of their drug. Up to now, the elder population has had little power to insist on more accurate information—we believe the time has come to change the paradigm. We will discuss specific examples, like the use of statins, in chapter 3. These examples are among the issues the aging population must think about and understand if they are to appropriately manage their health care. Inappropriate use of prescription drugs is also partly to blame for driving up the costs of health care and health insurance.

At a time when the health care system often fails us, insurance companies and health maintenance organizations are really Fortune 500 corporations lining the pockets of government bureaucrats and company CEOs, our population is more rotund and less active, and pharmaceutical companies are bombarding us with advertising to lure us into taking pills and potions for maladies we never knew existed (and likely do not have), we offer a different way to think about life. We are firmly convinced that life must be enjoyed to the fullest up to the end and that the path to thriving requires us to push aside much of medicine and the medical bureaucracy as we have known it and replace it with a vision of the future and the good things life offers us when we aggressively approach the elder phase of our life.

2

A Social Perspective

The impending crisis in Medicare and, more generally, the financing of health care for all in the United States, calls for clear articulation of what we, as a society, are about. Precisely what is our aim and how do we proceed to whatever goals we aspire? For sure, we must admit that there is no consensus as to what might characterize that aim, but that should not deter us from laying out the prime issues that must shape whatever we hope to do. Most important, this crisis cannot be addressed as a narrow "health care" issue. What we must talk about is the quality of life for all residents of the United States, including elders.

This book is our attempt to address this matter and it reflects our experiences and values. In no way is it intended to convey that this is the only or the best prescription, but we do hope it is coherent and consistent and will contribute to the debate.

What Do We Mean By Health Care For Elders?

To be a bit more precise: What kind of access ought elders have to the myriad of remedies and treatments that are now and will be in the future available for the treatment of the physical and mental ailments that beset all humanity? To a certain degree, answering that question entails recommendations for research on new technology oriented to the problems of aging, but for the greater part it concerns the appropriate delivery of what is generally available to the public as a whole.

Social versus Private Goals

In modern Western society there is widespread acceptance of a predominant public interest and, therefore, an acceptance of the appropriate role for a designated collective (government) that functions in an array of activities to fulfill those public interests; e.g., defending the nation, maintaining highways, fighting fires, educating children, and ensuring food safety. This has not necessarily taken the form of direct government activity—often, public regulation of private collective activities has been the approach. On the other hand, there are uncountable activities for which the consensus is that purely private actions are appropriate; e.g., while present law demands that the operation of a motor vehicle requires having liability insurance in most states, probably no one believes the inclusion of collision insurance in a policy is a matter of public concern. Hence, we must take a stand on what is the public (or social) interest in providing health care for elders.

So, how do we rationalize that balance? One way would be to rely on a libertarian prescription for private health care; i.e., let each individual (or family unit) take responsibility for obtaining access to the health care they desire. Why not allow consumers and the private free market to assemble the options in concert, leaving it to the responsible individual to decide what costs and risks are to be taken? The answer is simple: unlike grizzly bears, humans are a social species. (As a political aside, it should be no surprise that the "mama grizzly" is the chosen symbol of a current political faction in the United States. On the other hand, selecting a donkey for a political party is not very encouraging.) Whether or not one accepts the evolutionary view that social behavior was a key factor in the success of Homo sapiens, it is clear that group association has been a dominant feature of all we know about our past. This observation is not to demean the private individual—we are not akin to an ant species and, rightly, we hold in highest esteem the outstanding individual and give greatest praise to individual accomplishments in whatever field of endeavor. But, it is precisely because we humans are such a mix of the individual and the social that questions about appropriate access to health care are so perplexing.

There are at least two reasons why the public interest impinges on health care. First is the social response—instinctively we are moved by the plight of fellow humans we see in distress. When an individual or family is beset by a tragic accident or sickness, there frequently emerges a strong community response to provide assistance. This is highly commendable, but also sad—a system that requires this voluntary humanitarian response is hardly one in which to take pride. Even sadder is the knowledge that many such predicaments do not carry the emotion-evoking weight needed to capture voluntary action. We do acknowledge, however, that society has not been completely derelict. The social instinct has forced at least minimal access to be available to all in the form of the Emergency Room.

Second is the understanding that the well-being of all in society is heavily dependent on the robustness of the health of our fellow citizens. There is little reason to believe there is not widespread acceptance of this concept in general.

The nature of this dependence for elders differs from that of the younger cohorts of the population. There are few who are middle age and older that are unaware of the devastating emotional and economic price that must be paid by untold numbers of caregivers and supporters of the seriously ill or poorly functioning elders. This toll on individuals creates an aggregate that constitutes a high cost to society as a whole. The days of our grandparents—when the relatively small "very old" population could be looked after by extended family in a stable social environment—are long gone. Today there are ever-stronger reasons for a social response.

What Are the Ingredients of Normal Healthy Aging?

To address a sensitive and controversial issue at the outset: in considering the public interest, we decidedly are not advocates of indefinite "life extension" as a goal. In our view, the philosophical, ethical, and economic questions raised by the prospect of indefinite life expectancy presently are well beyond the capacity of a reasonable societal response. To state it clearly, we believe there is no social entitlement to indefinite life extension. In a recent web blog on the predictions, prospects, and promises of technology for producing indefinitely long life spans, one comment by an observer (probably an elder or approaching that) stood out as particularly astute: "I'd settle for a cure for hemorrhoids." We might do well to adopt that as the watchword for our position.

There is one aspect of life extension that is relevant to our considerations. In 1912, premature death was both a private and social concern. At present, it can be argued that premature death remains a private problem but not a social one. If anything, it might be argued that "post-mature" death is the emerging social problem.

What is premature death? For the private concern, the definition of premature is in the eye of the beholder. It is almost a mantra for our generation to assert that we do not want to reach the age or stage of disability that we witnessed in our parents, and others but neither do we want to expire right away. To die tomorrow would be premature. It is rather like giving up smoking—"One more cigarette won't hurt . . ." or, from the musical Annie, "Tomorrow is always a day away." We cannot hope to resolve those dilemmas here.

What should constitute premature death from a social perspective? We propose the following: When an individual has completed his or her "fiduciary" responsibilities to family, to other dependents, and to society, then death ought not to be considered premature by society. However, since individual circumstances are not appropriate to public policy, a simpler standard must serve. For lack of a better number, we suggest the wisdom of the authors of the Old Testament of the Bible—three score and ten as a reasonable marker. To be clear, we are not arguing that life beyond 70 years is undesirable for individuals (if that were the case, perhaps we should not be here to make these proposals). We are arguing that the public interest does not call for intervention at this stage as a social goal per se. We also argue that life beyond 70 years of age should be guided by issues of personal comfort, not by proposals related to life extension.

Rather, we advocate as a social aim a lesser version of the end expressed by Oliver Wendell Holmes in his poem, The One Hoss Shay. It would be nice to believe a logical end, as for the Shay, could exist, but in the modern world of technology that is not probable. We are all inexorably pushed toward indefinite life extension. A useful term for our overall concept could be "Healthy Normal Aging." Our touchstone is that absent heroic medical/technical intervention there is a plausible distribution of ages at which death is normal.

That the spread in that distribution is quite large does not negate the concept.

Healthy Normal Aging would then assert: After the marker age, the time is up; applying spectacular new technology and heroic measures is no longer a social responsibility. Now, if the social costs were known and low, our position could change. But they are not known and, almost certainly, they will not be low. In our view, that is the crisis in health care for elders. Acknowledging that there are higher-priority social needs is a must.

The focus we propose for Healthy Normal Aging is elimination or amelioration of those conditions that prevent aging from being a satisfactory path to a soft landing. That does mean much more than access to health care narrowly defined.

We propose our own list of ingredients within a concept of Healthy Normal Aging. Its overarching theme is independence. But by that we do not mean stand-alone self-gratification. Rather we mean the ability freely to be, to do, and to participate in—that is, to function responsibly as an adult. That entails many factors, some admittedly extremely difficult to bring about. Healthy Normal Aging is a combined responsibility of the individual and society. Its precepts include:

1. Responsibilities
    Remaining informed
    Taking only what we're due, individually and collectively; being responsible to those who follow
    Avoiding "divide and conquer" mentality; not allowing ourselves to be exempt from the burdens that subsequent generations will be asked to carry in any reform program

2. Economic security
    Assuring an appropriate minimum social standard of income for all
    Taking individual responsibility for what is desired above that minimum
    Functioning securely in this rapidly changing world of technology and finance

3. Viable independent living
    Having access to services necessary to maintain a home
    Having mobility in the local community

4. Family and friends
    Maintaining access to family and friends
    Having something to say, being listened to and taken seriously, and telling your story

5. Living in the community and greater world
    Interacting with others having common interests
    Taking advantage of opportunities to help others
    Having access to institutions and services like libraries, social clubs, and gyms
    Having the ability to participate in recreational activities: travel near and far, swim, paint a landscape, pick berries, grow plants, go to a baseball game, ride a bicycle, take grandchildren to the playground, etc.
    Having access to, understanding of, and facility in dealing with the world out there
    Having an ability and opportunity to make our views known

Avoiding past presumptions on what must constitute the "good" life; i.e., being pigeonholed

6. Physical comfort
   Having access to relief from chronic pain and discomfort with minimal side effects
   Having assurance that bodily deterioration and ailments are cared for in a compassionate setting
   Maintaining the ability to hold, to sit, to reach, to walk, to climb stairs
   Maintaining the ability to savor the world, particularly good vision and hearing
   Identifying and treating chronic debilitating diseases

7. Mental health
   Treating and curing dementia and Alzheimer's disease
   Maintaining self-esteem and a feeling of positive contribution
   Avoiding and treating depression
   Altering the prevailing image of elder "decline"—a problem of isolation, not aging

8. Transitions
   Receiving tender loving care in moving to more dependent living
   Finally, having a soft landing (a comfortable exit, rather than repetitive preservation by means of heroic interventions)

There is little about quantity in Healthy Normal Aging—it is about quality. We must decide as individuals and as a society what sort of a commitment we are prepared to make. Elders are increasing in numbers but are not the only members of society. Even if our will should be there, the dictates of economics must govern; we cannot do everything for everyone.

Given the current political environment, the preeminent question in this nation is: How should we apportion the response between the private and societal roles? And, as a corollary: To what degree ought the societal response be governmental or voluntary? Here, I leave these as open questions. In chapter 11, Summarizing Recent Proposals to Reform Medicare, and appendix B: A Conceptual Societal Health Program for Elder, we offer our views on the matter.

What We Need to Do
As Individuals

3

Frequent Minor Problems of Elders

Every aging person must deal with many persistent, but minor, problems. The short list includes tinnitus; cataracts; muscle and joint weakness and resulting instability; general pain from muscle loss and slower healing; memory loss; depression due to changing societal roles, fear of incontinence and loss of mobility and anxiety due to all of the above.

We think now of the quote from the movie *Monty Python and the Holy Grail*—in the film, there is a scene where victims of a plague epidemic are being thrown onto a cart and a tiny voice from the bottom of the pile cries out: "I'm not dead yet . . . I'm not dead yet." One of the men piling the bodies on the cart responds with hostility, "Don't worry—you will be soon!" That is the way all too many of us elders feel all too frequently. Here, we provide some hopeful advice for the future.

The main thing to keep in mind is that you are neither almost dead nor are you likely in need of medical treatment. Your life will be greatly enhanced and your healthy longevity improved by: taking some well-considered pain-relief medication; exercising; accepting tinnitus and adding sound diversion to your environment (sound machines that create white noise or background noise);

understanding intention tremor (the tremor of muscle imbalance as one intends to make a move—it is not Parkinson's disease); participating in creative activities like writing, gardening, making music, drawing, etc.; stimulating memory via crossword puzzles and complex card games; and, perhaps most important, avoiding medication other than those for specific and defined symptoms. The pain-relief medication should be in the form of well-tested opiates, not nonsteroidal anti-inflammatory drugs (NSAIDs) that you probably do not need. Effective pain-relief medications require a prescription and medical supervision; they are for improving life quality, not for remedying or removing a specific disease process. In other words, by eliminating the often chronic physical aches and pains that accompany the aging process, day-to-day life will be greatly improved.

As we will discuss later, one reason not to use NSAIDs is that when we are over 70 years old, support is needed for increased healing via natural inflammation and metabolic processes, not by inhibiting these mechanisms. It may be a challenge to obtain a low dose of codeine or morphine—not because they do not help but because physicians fear they will get into trouble if some patients become addicted to the drugs or that some may try to sell the drugs to make extra cash to supplement their fixed income. In order to obtain such medications, it is likely that you will be required to sign a statement to account for the drugs used (or unused).

On the surface, it may appear that a newer drug called oxycodone is useful or perhaps not as harmful as other opiates. We are discouraged from recommending it for two reasons. First, oxycodone is no more effective than morphine derivatives but it appears to be much more addictive and requires more careful medical supervision during its use. Second, it appears that oxycodone has been at the center of criminal drug activity across state lines. Recently, 200 physicians identified in Florida were apparently reimbursed with health care funds of up to $25,000 per day when they wrote prescriptions for the distribution huge quantities of such drugs. The drugs were prescribed to drug dealers for bogus illnesses and the drugs, after being purchased at local pharmacies, ended up in the hands of drug addicts all over the eastern United States. The physicians and the drug dealers involved made considerable profits from this illegal activity, but the Florida state attorney decided it was too costly to identify and prosecute the criminals.

We hope that low-dose morphine-derived pain medication will be more easily available to all people over 70 years of age. The greatest stumbling block preventing this is the necessity of state or federal regulatory control of the companies manufacturing and selling the drugs to ensure quality, as well as oversight of the pharmacies dispensing them (allowing for unethical practices by a small number of greedy physicians). This is the kind of issue where elders and advocates should make their voices heard in the United States Congress.

One of the challenges for elders is to establish a balance between maintaining some vibrant life activities in the face of increased real or perceived movement limitations. This problem of "decline" in physical and mental abilities will be discussed in a subsequent chapter of the book, but we assert that "decline" is a flawed concept. We now know that the perception of decline is not a result of the aging process but of two distinct life changes that affect us all. First, elders become increasingly isolated following retirement and their children leaving home (often to start their own families in geographically distant locales). In addition, our circle of friends tends to diminish because of illness or death and geographic relocation after retirement.

Second, there is a natural change in muscle biochemistry over time that leads to a loss of muscle mass—this means, for example, that an athlete cannot run as fast when older as when young, but this is due to some natural protective mechanisms the body employs to prevent age-related cell destruction.

John Cotton, the author of chapter 2, is an avid cyclist. He has noted that his comfortable riding speed has declined over time—from 18 mph at age 45, to 12 mph at age 76. In addition, his heart rate during exercise actually went down from 200 beats per minute (bpm) at age 45, to 175 bpm at age 76. He thought these numbers were evidence of decline but, in fact, they reflect valuable metabolic changes in aging individuals. They are signs of change that should be noted but do not necessarily indicate any need for medical intervention. John continues to ride daily as part of his aggressively healthy lifestyle.

Gardening activities, cycling, participating in the household and helping with children, preparing meals, shopping, attending cultural events, reconciling one's check book, paying bills, and planning for enjoyable outings and vacations must be included as a normal part of life—not focusing predominantly on your health.

4

Maintaining an Active and Fulfilling Lifestyle

There are many ways to remain active in those years following a fulltime career and after children have established lives of their own. An important feature of aging is the loss of muscle mass. Regular exercise cannot entirely halt this process. This means that if a 75-year-old is inactive for several weeks, it will take months to restore the body to the level that existed prior to the inactive period. Clearly, daily activity including exercise is essential. In their book, Burton and Hall recommend 30 minutes per day as a reasonable target. If pain control is necessary to maintain this activity level, it should be in the form of the lowest dose of anti-pain medication possible rather than mood-elevating drugs or NSAIDs. Daily exercise is the key to aging aggressively. My wife and I keep an advertisement from a Swiss journal attached to our refrigerator as a daily reminder of the need for exercise. The ad features a female elder stretching with her leg above her head and a caption that reads, "Our customers are young and agile, no matter how old they are!"

Other minor problems of aging include disturbances in sleep patterns, easy fatigability, grumpiness or short temper (that may result from constant low-grade muscle or joint discomfort), intestinal problems of occasional diarrhea or constipation, and lethargy in the absence of clearly defined goals or responsibilities for the day or the week. When discussed with a physician, any of these disturbances might lead to a suggestion for sleep medication, mood elevators, anti-diarrheal or constipation medication, stimulants for fatigue, or vitamins. Rather than medication, we recommend that joint and muscle aches be dealt with first by insuring the right amount of physical activity each day. Exercise generates endorphins that improve our mood and overall peace of mind.

Sleep disturbances can be dealt with by adjusting our schedules to read or do calming activities prior to going to sleep or during the time we are undesirably awake. For example, some people have trouble falling asleep when they get into bed; some others awaken at midnight or 4:00 a.m. A publication that is fun to read but not a "page-turner" or a simple crossword puzzle or Sudoku may help. Usually 30 minutes to an hour should get your sleep mechanism back into gear. One should also be sure to drink adequate amounts of water to avoid dehydration—this is a frequently overlooked problem among elders.

To ensure a good night's sleep, it is also a good idea to avoid eating a heavy evening meal or drinking excessive amounts of alcohol. Having a light meal at 6:00 p.m. or 7:00 p.m. (a broiled chicken breast and vegetables, or fruit and cheese, or a delicious salad) accompanied by a glass of wine should satisfy most appetites without weighing on us later in the evening.

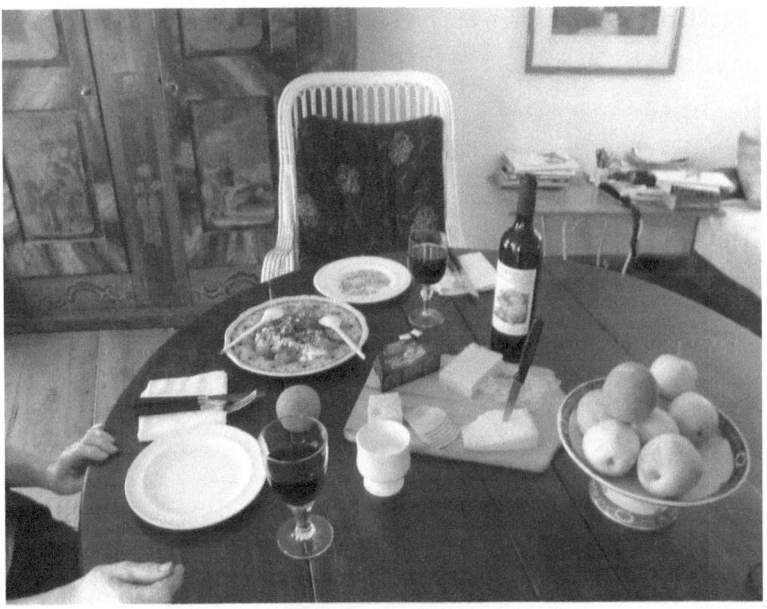

Figure 1. The author's typical evening meal.

Intestinal problems should be evaluated to identify the most likely cause. Excessive morning sympathetic nervous system activity leading to loose stools each day is common. The cause may not be easily defined, but the problem requires additional hydration and can often be solved by increasing water intake. Constipation can usually be remedied by drinking prune juice and increasing fiber intake at meals; for example, adding oatmeal or a whole grain cereal to breakfast every morning and more fruit and vegetables throughout the day.

Fatigue and grumpiness can be helped by an afternoon nap and adopting a general sense of good humor. Having children in the house can help provide humor but there must be ground rules about the amount of rowdiness and noise that is acceptable. For such occasions when children are present, a good book of jokes or riddles or games that everyone can participate in can be fun to share.

To ensure a sense of purpose, scheduled daily activities are essential. Simple chores like shopping for food and other essentials, daily walks, attending cultural events, lunch dates with friends and family members, gardening, practicing an instrument, or learning another language, etc., should all be part of a daily routine and will contribute to a fulfilling lifestyle.

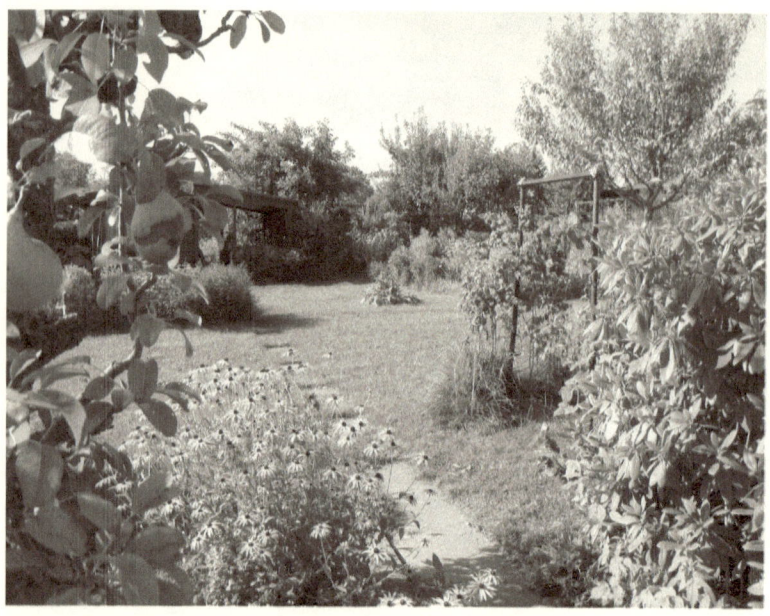

Figure 2. The author's garden/farm.

By the way, gardening is not a new idea for keeping fit. Here is a photo of John Cotton's grandfather in his garden in 1964. At the age of 90 years, he looked fit!

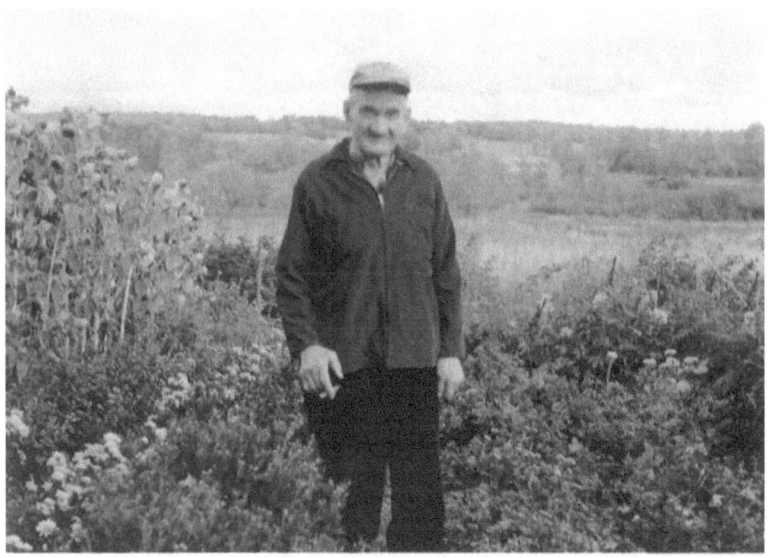

Figure 3 JFC's Grandfather at age 90 in his garden.

As we age, often surrounded by younger people, we are sometimes asked to try something new. If we refuse, or we attempt the action or suggestion poorly, then the old phrase you can't teach an old dog new tricks is often applied. There are several things wrong with that conclusion. First, there is limited data to support the statement that older dogs (or humans) have difficulty learning. Most cognitive or physical decline with aging is based on diminished environmental input, not self-deterioration. Second, the refusal to learn something is more likely a choice to avoid the experience or activity.

We have all been asked to try a long list of things, including hang gliding, mountain climbing, eating a new preparation of a food we are not fond of, using a cell phone, taking recreational drugs, swimming with sharks, "texting" to our grandchildren, etc. Based on our experiences, we may balk at such suggestions, but can we learn something new?

Let us discuss the data to support or reject the notion of poor learning skills among elders. We believe the notion of old dogs/new tricks has more to do with sensory deprivation or lack of interest than brain dysfunction. Unfortunately, most of the studies on older people have been done in care centers, not in the market place. As an aside, as a renegade statistician, the author has said that the market place is statistically a better place to be standing than in a hospital ward. The chance of dying among people standing in the market is perhaps 1 in 1,000; in a hospital it is 1 in 50—the clear message here is, stay out of the hospital!

We all have fun testing our memory as we grow older. It has been stated that short-term memory goes first. Our argument to that is obvious—the brain has a finite amount of space, so as we age there is less available space because of all the stuff that has been collected over the years. (Admittedly, there is a neuropsychological limit, not a neurophysical one since the brain has almost endless electrical impulse interaction potential). The new stuff tries to get in but there just is not enough room. . . .

The other argument is that memory has to have something to connect to or build on—like the famous learning tree. The author's wife can remember almost any word in English, Latin, Italian, French, or German because she was a language teacher and a linguist, but she has trouble remembering whether she purchased all of the items we need for lunch as we sit down to eat. The author, on the other hand, cannot remember how to spell a word (to be fair, he never could), but he has no trouble remembering what he and his wife decided during breakfast to have that day for lunch.

5

Obtaining Appropriate Physical and Mental Support, Health Advice and Nursing Care

We have all attempted to find a solution to a perceived health problem from a person other than our physician, or by an alternative rather than standard treatment. The phrase "self-medication" indicates a process whereby a patient takes medication without a physician's intervention. This term covers a great number of methods for self-treatment, including taking medication prescribed for an illness in a family member, taking the advice of a friend who recalls having had similar symptoms, and purchasing something seen on an infomercial or advertisement.

On the other hand, we might get advice from paramedical personnel like pharmacists, pharmacy assistants, nurses, or practitioners of alternative forms of medicine. Paramedical personnel may be quite well-informed about medications and their use. Pharmacists, in particular, often know more about the drugs being dispensed than the physicians. The reality is that paramedical personnel provide a large part of health care worldwide and, generally, do a good job. The issue, therefore, is not how to better regulate drug distribution but how to better educate those who end up in such an important position in the institution of health care delivery.

Who to Turn to for Health Advice

In a related context, this author was involved in discussions with regulatory authorities in the United Kingdom concerning over-the-counter (OTC) availability of an anti-fungal drug for treating athlete's foot and whether unsupervised use (or overuse) could lead to emerging anti-microbial resistance. While reviewing literature related to this issue, strong opinions emerged regarding pharmacy availability of antibiotics but very little evidence that this practice contributed to the problem.

So, does over-the-counter availability of antibiotics lead to an increase in anti-microbial resistance? Although opinions on this issue are strong, the data are weak. Antibiotic resistance emerges among immune-compromised patients in hospitals, not among healthy people with self-limiting diseases in pharmacies. The argument presented to health care regulators in the UK was that requiring a prescription for treatment of athlete's foot had a far worse effect on health care economics and physician resources than the perceived beneficial effect of preventing emerging drug resistance.

On this topic, the greatest attention has been focused on the activities of physicians. For example, one major report identified that the most frequent source of antibiotic misuse was by a busy physician consulted by a patient with a respiratory illness. The report indicated that inappropriate antibiotic prescribing by a busy physician was responsible for over 90% of inappropriate antibiotic use in the United Kingdom. This same high frequency of antibiotic use for minor respiratory illness has also been recorded in the United States.

In addition, another report indicated that a pharmacist was more likely to provide an inappropriate antibiotic than was a pharmacy assistant. One could conclude that the higher up on the health care ladder one is, the more likely they are to contribute to the misuse of antibiotics! It appears, therefore, that the real question is not how to regulate medication distribution better, but how to be sure the best information on the issue is provided at all levels of health care distribution. Indeed, in the opinions voiced in the House of Lords Report referred to above, antibiotic use or misuse must be viewed as a cultural event, not a medical, scientific event. Detailed exploration of this cultural event is needed.

There are other concerns about prescription medications being distributed by paramedical personnel. To avoid the potential of a profit motive influencing the prescribing process in the United States, rules were established in the 1950s so that the person who prescribed a medication was not permitted to also dispense the drug—that led to a major change in drug availability in the United States. Rather than requiring the two-step procedure current in the United States, we believe it might be possible that educating, monitoring, and supervising prescribing patterns in pharmacies could be a more direct and less costly way to prevent problems from emerging.

Is it a reasonable approach to educate pharmacists to make diagnoses of mild or common complaints (those requiring only non-prescription drugs), or must the process be regulated? As a realistic approach to health care, the former must be seriously considered. One might even consider having a physician backup available by telephone for questions that arise in a pharmacy. This approach is currently being done in pharmacies throughout the United States to administer flu vaccine; many other vaccines are currently administered in travel clinics with a physician "backup" (by phone or internet) present.

Another aspect to consider is the financial impact created by patients avoiding a physician's office for diagnoses and prescriptions. On one hand, using a pharmacy for diagnosing illness and providing non-prescription medication is cheaper for both the health care system and the patient. On the other, the well-trained physician is bypassed after having invested considerable time and money to prepare for this task. In some instances, physicians feel forced to prescribe a drug to justify the expense the patient has paid for advice, or to ensure a happy patient who will likely return, or from fear of legal action if the untreated patient's illness worsens.

There is, occasionally, a more sinister side to the writing of prescriptions by physicians. As reported in chapter 3, quoting a Florida newspaper, unscrupulous physicians have been discovered writing unnecessary or inappropriate prescriptions for patients in order to defraud health care funding agencies. Such practices have included prescriptions paid for by Medicare and Medicaid. For example, a patient (with a real or fictional name) is given a prescription for some medication, then the documentation that the prescription was written is submitted to the relevant funding agency for reimbursement to the physician for the time and the expertise required. Of course, this is illegal, but the unscrupulous physician is tempted to double or triple his income simply by writing prescriptions. This is a problem that requires greater oversight and regulation but, unfortunately, is likely underfunded in a shortsighted effort to reduce costs. Perhaps these agencies should consider subtracting a payment for each prescription written over a certain number—OK, that may be impossible, but it is worth thinking about.

Is it appropriate and is it good medicine for a local pharmacist to replace the family physician, as has already occurred in some poor countries? Would the cost of drugs be lower or higher without physician intervention? Who would determine diagnosis accuracy? These questions must be answered, and then they will require a socially sensitive, medically appropriate response. Regional and national health care issues will have to be considered, but the right answers might result in a significant benefit to patients' quality of life and financial status.

One of the dangers each of us faces as we age is that questions are raised about the cost of medications and services we receive in relation to the contribution each of us makes to society. These questions have often been hidden in the fine print, but they are there. In the politics of worldwide application of health care, government providers have often turned to the statistical tool termed "cost-benefit ratio." This analysis determines the cost of a new treatment and then calculates the financial benefit of a death prevented by its use.

The use of cost-benefit analysis has been mentioned many times over the years when considering the proposed use of cholera vaccine or rotovirus vaccine, and it has been a part of the basis in assessing the use of meningococcal vaccine in sub-Sahara Africa. In each case, program planners considered how the cost would compare to the health care budgets available in the countries most likely to need the vaccine, and how much cost would be added to ongoing vaccine programs.

Hidden in such questions is the bureaucratic issue of how much the present ineffective program of caring for ill, dying, or dead people costs. By asking the question in this way, one clearly finds that the present ineffective program is cheaper and that the added expense of vaccines does not result in new cost savings in the workforce, does not ensure greater consumer availability, nor does it reduce costs for the ill and dying. Therefore, it should not be done! There is little doubt that the most effective means of keeping health care costs low is to do nothing and promote the idea of sudden death—that is the cheapest method of health care.

It is, indeed, fortunate that such calculations were not used at the turn of the 20th century when health care officials were deciding how to establish tuberculosis control programs, develop vaccines against tetanus and diphtheria, and identify typhoid carriers in Europe and the United States. The cost of polio and smallpox campaigns would bring loud negative votes from the cost-benefit calculators of today.

One can search the literature in vain (see one exception below) to find the answer to the underlying question: How much is a life worth? That question should be answered first, then a determination made on how to find the capacity and funds to ensure that a premature death is prevented.

First, let us refer to a study done in Sweden several years ago in which government regulators, using a cost-benefit analysis, tried to decide whether a longterm and rather expensive drug for treating aged patients with bone marrow cancer, or *agnogenic myeloid metaplasia*, was worth the expense. It was, indeed, an expensive therapy costing $50,000 to $100,000 per year. Then, perhaps for the first time, authorities tackled the question of how much a Swedish elder was worth. They came to the incredible decision that each Swede was actually worth $50,000 to $100,000 so they approved the drug for use!

If we come to the same conclusion that each one of us is worth the expenditure of, perhaps, $20,000 to $30,000 per year to prevent premature death in parts of the Western world (other than in

Sweden), and perhaps $1,000 to $2,000 in Africa, then let us start our debate on the measures to prevent death. Of course, we will soon come to the problem that, using present rules as indicated above, a life in a relatively rich country is worth more than a life in Africa.

Maybe it is time for us to face this question, too. Premature death may be difficult to define, but certainly infant mortality counts, as does death during epidemics of infectious diseases. How much should be spent to prevent premature deaths specifically among elders (as opposed to other premature deaths)?

A physician in Switzerland recently complained that because of the national health insurance approach, those that smoke or become obese should have a higher insurance premium, much as is required of airplane pilots for life insurance. As the physician researched the issue he learned that smokers and obese people tend to die suddenly of heart attacks or of untreatable lung cancer, so they are actually less expensive for the health care system than those of us who get old with chronic diseases of the bones, joints, and brain. The physician considered starting a campaign to encourage smoking and weight gain in order to reduce health care insurance payments—but then he realized that the young Swiss people who do not read or think are solving the problem of health care costs themselves: they smoke, they are overweight, and they die at a younger age with less cost to the health care system.

Perhaps we should think as lawyers. Lawyers working with actuaries have been able to establish a price for death following airline disasters. The main difference between death from an airline crash and death in a village in a poor country or in a nursing home in the United States is that the lawyers know exactly who to sue for the lost life in a plane crash. It would seem that we need only determine who should be sued in the case of an infant's death due to respiratory or gastrointestinal disease, or an elder patient's death in a hospital where care has been determined inadequate. We could start by suing the government for inadequate regulatory oversight or the pharmaceutical companies (as was recently done to the tobacco industry) or the World Health Organization (WHO) for not ensuring proper distribution of health care. The list could grow very long. One could also begin a system of international health care insurance for companies, hospitals, and governments. Each potentially preventable death would lead to a payment of $1,000 to $30,000 by the health system within which the death occurred. The insurance companies would collect premiums from those most likely to be liable for the premature death. Thus, not only would funds become available where needed to prevent the next death but the payment of premiums would be by those who, by their inaction, allow the problem in the first place. It is true that this would become a very large industry, perhaps surpassing the present defense industry.

The important question is how can these complex problems of expensive health care and exorbitant insurance payments be solved? The answer is clear: a minimum acceptable standard of health care and nutrition must be guaranteed everywhere. Achieving this goal will require very clever and creative planners. Our point here is that until we remove the hidden institutionalized guidelines that accept the status quo and fail to measure how much a human life is worth in our society, we cannot begin to answer the question of how to do it better. All things are possible once we get rid of this cost-effectiveness mentality.

One of the main reasons that the elder population is growing is due to improved access to the technical advances in rapid amelioration of health care problems. These advances are not only in the direct application of drugs (for example, thrombolytic therapy

[tPA] to break up or dissolve blood clots for stroke), but in rapid care and resolution of blocked cardiac and carotid arteries, rapid care for spinal and hip injuries, reduced in-hospital time that has prevented blood clots and nosocomial infections, and cancer (specifically by early diagnoses of breast, prostate, and colon cancers). So a key feature of care for elders is speedy access to the correct procedures at the right time, currently paid for by Medicare (in the United States) or other health insurance.

Physical and Mental Support

In cases where technical methods alone are no longer useful or are inadequate, the big challenge that elders and their families must address is when to call in community-based health care assistance. Generally, family and close friends provide the first stage of assisted care. This is a wonderful and ancient tradition that must be supported in every way possible. Eventually, however, professional and organizational assistance is likely to be needed. The assistance may include meal services, bed and toilet assistance, ambulation activity, nursing home or hospital transfer, or providing an assisted exit-from-life program (called "Exit" or *Dignitas*, currently in Switzerland). An alternative is offered in the state of Oregon, as well. This chapter will provide you with some of the details needed for each of these steps.

Your primary care provider must play an important role in providing referrals or discussing how to obtain the various services you may need. Here, we provide some information about how you and your care provider may best be able to obtain necessary services. Going forward, we hope you can transfer these details into your own community, county, or state. It is very important to realize the necessity of planning for your longterm future early in life. Your family must be included in these discussions and decisions since they will be impacted by your choices as well. It is apparent that some community and government lobbying will be necessary by all of us to ensure our future care.

Many elders require rehabilitation or physical therapy for acute or chronic injuries that impair their ability to function at a premium level in society. They also require rapid and affordable access to physical and cognitive exercise facilities that provide expert physical therapists, speech therapists, nurses, social workers, and physicians. These rehabilitation centers exist, but are not necessarily available in the rapid and affordable manor required. Here we provide an example of how to identify a rehabilitation program near your home. We will use the state of Florida as an example.

The best route to locating services is to use the internet to explore the Florida Health Care Program at www.myflorida. com (most states, counties, and cities have websites with such information). Look up the centers closest to your home and see what local community support may be available to help ensure rapid and complete attention for your specific needs. For example, in Martin County, Florida, retirement centers, recreational facilities, physical therapy clinics, and nursing homes are all available. Once you have identified an appropriate site, you will have to telephone them to determine important details like the cost of physical therapy or exercise programs and how long the waiting list is to begin treatment; whether they are certified by state and medical organizations; whether Medicare, part B or C, or Medicaid insurances are accepted and what type of private insurance can be used. A referral from your primary health care provider is often needed and, of course, your health care provider can give you information based on his or her experience regarding the center you have selected. An appointment at the center will also be important to determine if it fits your needs (not your physician's, your insurer's, or the center's needs). After careful review, it is a pleasure for this author to report that the services provided by assisted living facilities, physical therapy centers, and nursing homes in Florida are among the best examples of health care in the United States.

All of these services require each individual's scrutiny and consideration. They are usually private, for-profit institutions, which means that, except for those receiving Medicaid, they are funded by out-of-pocket payments by the elder or by his or her private insurance. These facilities are often state regulated and receive appropriate review and supervision. Many appear to be customer directed and they rely on their customers to spread the word regarding their quality of services, care, and cost.

After careful research for this book, the author must state that his own profession (physician), his previous employer (the pharmaceutical industry), government plans (Medicare and Medicaid, with their inadequate funding and supervision), insurance companies (with their focus on investor profits), and even university medical centers (that rely on federal and pharmaceutical company funding) have not come close to providing appropriate care to their patients in comparison to the professional industry committed to it.

In Martin County, even the cost of $2,500 to $5,000 per month for a room or small apartment with meals, library facilities, transportation for outings, and daily physical activities appears reasonable. Thus, an elder with a pension or social security and investments of approximately $40,000 per year may receive excellent care. So, with some advanced planning, elders can have a comfortable, secure life in a sympathetic environment. From this perspective evolved the subtitle of this book, *How to Avoid the U.S. Health Care Crisis.*

Some other states we looked at were Massachusetts, where there are special agencies one can contact to help with sometimes overwhelming payment issues; and Ohio, where each county handles these services differently. Regardless of where you live, just as in Florida, you must contact each independent care center directly.

Nursing Care

Nursing care includes in-home services and various levels of care provided within facilities (from apartments to nursing homes). These can be easily accessed on the internet. To specifically find nursing homes, visit the web page www.medicare.gov. You must locate the state and county that interests you, and then identify the nursing homes relevant to your needs and location. There will be a map, the specific address, the size of the facility, and a rating system of 1 to 5. The rating system reflects only a few important items, such as the ratio of nurses to residents; fire standards; recent health inspection information; special quality measures; and any registered complaints. For information about availability of space, daily costs, insurance reimbursement eligibility, types of meals, bedside and/or dining room facilities, recreation areas, library programs, activities or social programs, or the type of patients accepted (mostly based upon ambulatory, mental, and physical status, etc.), you will have to telephone and visit the facility. This process is sufficiently complicated so you will have to determine your geographical location preference and the number of facilities you wish to explore before you begin your site visits. Most people prefer to be near their current home or near relatives. If other factors, such as cost or acceptance of insurance, require that you go further afield, be sure to check any state residency requirements for the facility you want to focus on.

You will also want to investigate the broad range of care providers in your neighborhood that offer a plethora of services. For example, in Florida you can review the Nursing Home Guide for what is termed "alternatives to nursing homes." These alternatives include adult care centers, adult family care centers, assisted living facilities, continuous care retirement centers, homemaker and companion agencies, nurse registries, and hospice programs. Each of these facilities will have to be seen in person to obtain the information key to your decisions regarding their usefulness to you or your family members. This author has been impressed by their professionalism.

Most important, it is vital that discussing the challenges of aging should no longer be taboo. The sooner we begin to discuss these issues with the younger generation, the more likely it is that solutions to these challenges will be found.

6

Educating Your Physician About Quality of Life Care

The first step in any educational process is to define the problem or question we need to learn about. This is a considerable challenge in health care because those involved in delivering care are generally considered (and often consider themselves) highly informed and able to provide their patients, medical association members, or political voting base with the best possible service. We are taking a risk here by pointing out that, in spite of most physicians being dedicated to truthful and informed service, there are major deficiencies in the information-and-delivery-of-service chain. Here we will provide sufficient examples to provoke us all to accept the need for a new mindset about health care delivery while not being too defensive about past failures.

Busy primary care physicians face a serious information transfer problem. This information gap results from several factors: often, many years have elapsed between medical school education and the present; annual medical conferences provide only a snapshot of current medical breakthroughs and are inadequate for keeping physicians up to date with the abundance of information needed to perform at the highest level; and there is little time for attendance at continuing education courses. The physician's failure to be "up to date" is due partly to the fact that the medical school curriculum of years ago did not cover issues important to quality of life today; and annual conferences focus predominantly on new technologies, not on the changing needs and attitudes about health management. As Burton and Hall pointed out in their book, the field of geriatrics did not even exist when they were in medical school. Much of the important information they conveyed to their readers was a result of years of dedicated experience.

As part of a new, and we believe necessary, mindset we would like to remind physicians and government officials of their duty to consider their new and important role in the health care industry. We are employing the commonly used phrase "health care industry" because this is the reality and the challenge each of us must face—health care has become an industry. This fact has good and bad features and we must spend the time to tease out the good, discard the bad, and devise a new method of delivering health care.

Here we ask the question and present a major premise of this book: Is health care really an industry like any other or is it an absolute need and right for all? We believe the concept of health care as "industry" must be removed and be replaced by the belief that health care is an absolute need and an absolute right.

Once we remove the word "industry" what exactly is universal health care? We believe that universal health care is about being interested in adequate nutrition for all people, the support for human dignity, and the assurance that each human being is able to maintain a reasonably functional, satisfying existence throughout their lifetime.

For some reason, society has decided that individual physicians should fulfill the challenge of providing universal health care—a totally unrealistic premise. At present, the physician is dependent on receiving timely medical information from organizations (like the pharmaceutical companies or physician practice associations) that are focused on their own bottom lines rather than on patients' inability to keep up with the escalating costs of care. And so it falls upon the physician to make up for the inadequate funding for patient health care needs and decide the future of his patient! This is the political reality and the political impossibility. Doctors have become victims of the health care industry just as have the patients.

There is only one answer to this mess—we must develop a system that allows physicians to re-educate themselves about how to help the patient so in need of medical, social, and quality of life care. The first step toward the solution is that each physician must become an activist and an advocate for his or her patients. The physician must enter the fray and be on the front line of revising health care insurance and pension plans. The physician must be an activist that requires a reasonable payment for patient services. Then, those same physicians must stand before the politicians and insist that the elder generation they represent will not tolerate further exclusion from the social-community process.

A major task for each person participating in the current health care environment is to take responsibility for telling their physician that they know they are likely to be misinformed by the pharmaceutically-driven media, the United States Food and Drug Administration (FDA), and the academic medical community, and then support—even insist on—change.

The following examples draw attention to two areas where misuse of language has prevented understanding of what is really going on and, as a result, prevented proper information exchange to allow us to solve the underlying problems. The areas focused on in this review are: 1) drug regulation, particularly by the FDA; and 2) language within pharmaceutical companies. There is a third area of language confusion and that is the complexity of the clinical trials research process. The clinical trials research process leads to the drugs you are advised to take in spite of the fact that it is seriously flawed. Due to the technical nature of the clinical trials process, we have included it in appendix A.

The FDA and Other Regulatory Agencies

The FDA has been a powerful force in the regulation of medicines and medical devices in the United States for over 50 years. During the past few decades, FDA policies have begun to be mirrored in many other parts of the world, most notably in Europe. The power of this agency and its expanding influence derived from several factors but, most important, from the desire of citizens to feel secure that a prescription medicine or an over-the-counter (OTC) drug has been properly tested and is safe for use. Due to a number of subtle mislabelling practices by the FDA, however, its role has expanded significantly, and at a tremendous cost, to include the entire process of regulating health care. The FDA promotes itself as a government agency established to "protect the public" but, using that definition, it has become a micromanager of all aspects of health care in our society. If each person knew what they had given up in the process of this evolution from drug safety to total drug control, we are certain there would be a request to take some of their own decision-making power back. Citizens should ask for a marked reduction in the power of the FDA and for a return to its role as a safety monitor rather than a drug controller.

High administrative costs, blunting drug development, and delays in drug and medical device availability have been well detailed in the book, *Hazardous to Our Health? FDA Regulation of Health Care Products* edited by Robert Higgs. Higgs describes that the FDA is not a body to ensure drug safety, but rather a law-enforcement and political body that has the goal to regulate, supervise, and partly determine the development, manufacture, advertising, and availability of all drugs.

Schematic Representation of the Regulatory Process for Drugs and Medical Devices

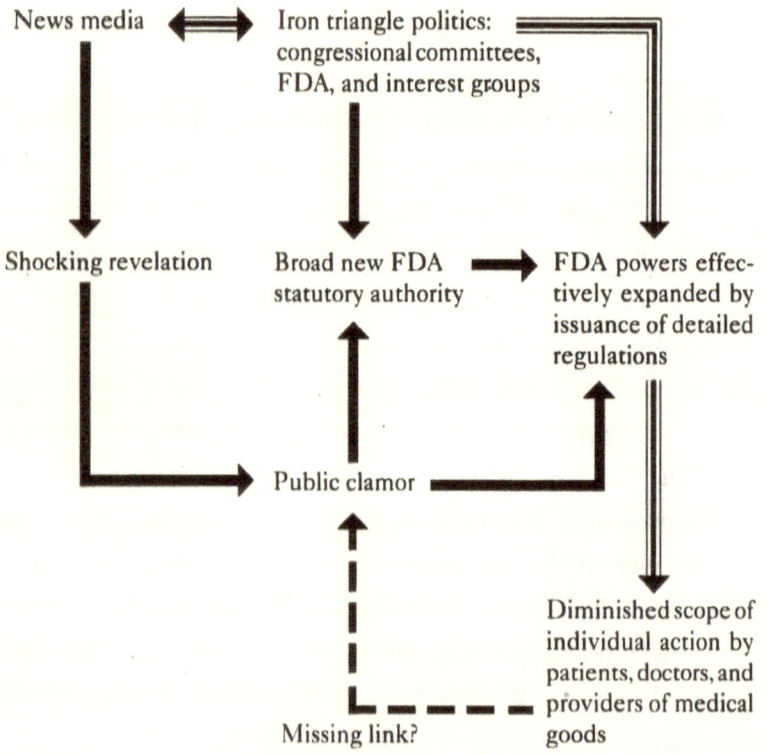

Figure 4. Diagram of FDA processes.

Just over the past 10 years, the cost of drug development has increased up to tenfold; as a result of the processes in place, delays in drug availability have increased two- to three-fold. This is only the tip of the iceberg, resulting from misguided trust in an agency originally established to supervise drug and device safety. There are numerous examples of how the change in operation of the FDA over the years has denied the public, including elders, numerous medications. Due to a number of bureaucratic obstacles, some people have had to wait for years to obtain a drug shown to be both effective and safe and widely used in other countries. Some drugs can only be obtained by going to Canada, which may be illegal, or by shopping on the internet.

The FDA has clearly misrepresented itself as an organization that ensures the safety of medicines and devices; in reality, the FDA is blocking and delaying creative drug development, increasing health care costs, and using government funds to pay the salaries of their army of statisticians, micromanagers, and bureaucrats. The agency involves itself in the composition of hospital clinical review boards, in the design of the clinical investigation process, and in manipulating the scientific direction of pharmaceutical research. This last point was made clear when a former FDA head told top executives of pharmaceutical companies to begin research on agents to inhibit the HIV virus or not bother bringing any drug for approval to the FDA. We may happen to share an enthusiasm for HIV research, but we cannot support the role of the FDA as a threatening force in the process. The FDA was doing the wrong thing under the wrong label.

Of course, regulatory agencies do not create deceptive practices alone. There is evidence that pharmaceutical companies and government finance offices participate as well, particularly in Europe. An example of pharmaceutical company participation putting up barriers to drug approval was seen recently in the new European Union rules regarding clinical trials necessary to register a drug already registered in one formulation—for example, a topical agent being available in a liquid solution instead of a cream.

Many years ago, a logical and inexpensive approach was required simply to prove that a new formulation did not alter tolerability, stability, or absorption of a drug. Since the active drug was already tested and registered, if no chemical alteration was demonstrated then the new formulation was registered. Now, major and costly drug development is required, as if a new formulation contains some new agent. This change requires action by a pharmaceutical company that costs anywhere from $500,000 to $10,000,000.

Surprisingly, the pharmaceutical companies supported this change, but why? This is a step in, what used to be called, "life-cycle management" of a drug. The pharmaceutical company's corporate financial and legal officers realized there was a far greater danger to their company than the added cost of a new study. That greater danger was future competition from companies who could make generic copies of their drug after the patent expired. The new rule makes it very expensive for a generic company to get into the game. So, who pays for this added cost? The public pays—fewer formulations of drugs are available and the potential reduction in drug costs is limited.

By misrepresenting its activities, the FDA has fooled the public into thinking that tax dollars are being used to protect them when, in fact, the FDA and other regulatory agencies have been denying the public potential life-saving medications marketed in a timely manner, resulting in increased health care costs. The approach taken by the regulatory agencies has had far reaching effects on the entire structure of the pharmaceutical industry. The new structure has led to the replacement of innovation with lots of paper, individual initiative with corporate regulatory-driven dictates, and personal responsibility with collective supervision. A health care disaster is in the making!

Pharmaceutical Companies

Perhaps the most important misuse of language concerning pharmaceutical companies is that they are referred to as—and are considered—pharmaceutical companies at all. In fact, almost all of the major pharmaceutical companies are actually financial holding companies that use their health care activities as a socially acceptable front. They can pretend to play a beneficial role in society while they are transferring funds from one corporate account or venture to another, down-sizing and merging, and maintaining the highest possible profit for their investors. (This activity is much the same process used by banks and insurance companies).

After pharmaceutical companies have been properly labeled as investor-driven holding companies, it is obvious why truly creative drug development is not an option in the pharmaceutical industry, particularly if it involves some extra financial investment. There is one sinister exception to this lack of creative development—the very small pharmaceutical research company that entices risk-taking investors to supply financial backing based on fantastic claims of innovation; then when it is about to be shown that the innovation is exaggerated, the company is sold to one of the above-mentioned financial holding companies at a nice profit to the few scientists that started the company. This sort of bootstrap capitalism may be the American way but it does not do much to provide effective and safe drugs for patients.

Let us assume, for purposes of discussion, that there are a few drug companies really interested in doing the basic research, followed by well-designed clinical trials to achieve the registration of a new chemical agent for use in patients to prevent or alter a disease process. Where are the mislabeling events occurring in such companies?

One of the most confusing terms, and one that has led to major problems, is research and development (or R and D, "R&D"). These two words characterize two distinct parts of a pharmaceutical company. The research is done by a group of "pre-clinical scientists." In order to successfully present a new chemical entity to management, this group must demonstrate the new entity's basic concepts in treating a disease, its efficacy in animals, and the toxicology profile in animals; then, research stops and development begins. This means that the decision to go forward with the drug has been made—it is a done deal. The only activity remaining in the clinical arena is development.

This simple development label means that it is inappropriate for anyone to ask new questions during the process of clinical trials because questions might hinder a rapid development process. For example, recombinant gene products, such as cytokines, are often human-host specific so all research must be done during the development phase, but the process was not designed for this. Testing drugs directly in humans is too complex and potentially unethical—therefore, it must be considered a part of the development phase of research. This is one reason that new products have so much trouble getting through the process. This approach is further supported by the methods used to design clinical trials. All contingencies regarding the action of a drug must be included in the protocol before the trial is started. If something important is observed during the trial, that observation may not be used in the present trial but must be the basis for a new trial to answer the question. But the pharmaceutical company has timelines for this development process and such a reexamination cannot fit their timelines; therefore, this clinical research activity must be ignored. This process does not occur because pharmaceutical companies are unreceptive to such observations, but because the regulatory agencies claim this is "massaging of data" and a potential bias. Thus, the term "development" in the process of clinical trials is fully supported by regulatory concepts. The process of research must be separate from the process of drug development. Would patients be interested in having significant observations that were made during the drug development process pursued? We think so.

A major problem for all of us—patients and physicians alike—is that the pharmaceutical industry is designed to make a profit for the pharmaceutical companies and dividends for investors. Therefore, one should not be surprised when a company develops a new drug and then paints the best possible picture of their newest product. To do this, some skewed or inaccurate statistical presentations are made at medical conferences attended by physicians, to physicians in their offices or in hospitals, and to you, the patients, by direct advertising. The problem of questionable drug advertising was emphasized recently by claims of fraud against academics that were putting their names on publications that were actually ghostwritten by writers employed by the pharmaceutical industry.

To this author, direct-to-patient advertising is particularly disturbing because those responsible for the advertising claim that important data is provided for the patient to discuss with his or her physician when, in fact, it rarely is. If one actually reads the second page of such advertising where the possible adverse effects are listed, no reasonable patient would want to take the drug or talk to a physician about it. The success of drug advertising relies on a beautiful picture of health on the first page, and microscopic-sized print on the second page. It is also interesting that, on the second page, the pharmaceutical company provides a telephone number to use in case you, the patient, cannot afford to pay for the drug. As it turns out, any payment assistance they provide is actually underwritten by the government—in fact, it is a Medicaid payment!

Also to Consider

Another important task is to be sure that your physician and his or her hospital associates are very clear concerning what you, the patient, want for your last few months of life. For example, you should not want intensive hospital care, but proper palliative care at home. You should not want cancer chemotherapy that may extend your life a few months if those few months are likely to be filled with tremendous cost in pain and suffering. You should not want preventative health care drugs tested on 30- to 60-year-olds that have not been proven to either extend or improve your quality of life. Here I cite an example of the problem of too much end-of-life health care directed at life extension as opposed to quality of life.

A man, a bit over 80 years old, was diagnosed as having cancer of the prostate. A well-respected specialist suggested that treatment would likely not be helpful and that at his advanced age the treatment was worse than the disease. In contrast, the man's primary Medicare (for-profit) HMO doctor urged aggressive treatment in the form of 27 radiation treatments (each treatment cost Medicare $1,100). Based on his longtime relationship with the primary physician, he agreed to the radiation. After nine treatments, he could not tolerate any more and ceased treatment. The treatment left him incontinent. A few years later, now dying of old age, he let himself be talked into a lung biopsy to see if the cancer "had spread" by his same for-profit HMO doctor who told him the biopsy would be nothing more than a "mosquito bite." Following the biopsy, he ended up in the ICU and, $170,000 later, he was in agony, had a horrible infection, and died miserably 6 months later.

Family members asked, "Why should 90% of our medical dollars be spent during the last six months of our lives and why should elders be tortured with treatments that are worse than their diseases? Why spend your last months in a hospital when you could have around-the-clock treatment at home? Why?"

The answer is that we all have to learn to say, "No!" to procedures such as radiation treatment if it has no hope of improving our condition; "No!" to invasive procedures like kidney dialysis or complex lung or heart surgical approaches that weaken us and decrease potential quality time in our own environment; "No!" to useless diagnostic procedures; "No!" to artificial feeding and hydration methods. A peaceful time at home with family and friends, supported by in-home assistants to keep us comfortable, should be our goal.

Your physician may have difficulty accepting your decisions because medical training has taught him or her to do everything possible to keep you alive, regardless of financial cost or discomfort. Unfortunately, as in the case of the for-profit Medicare-supported HMO, the physician may be benefiting financially from the decision to extend your life with various drugs or procedures. Despite your physician's point of view, sometimes one just has to say, "No!"

7

When Medications, Diagnostic
Tests and Procedures Are Needed
and When They Are Not

We will begin our discussion with the most useful and important medications for those over 65 years of age. We will assume that the ailments we refer to here were actually diagnosed by a physician and were found to be interfering with the patient's quality of life.

For example, if there is evidence of heart or renal insufficiency then fluid and salt management with diuretics are needed; if significant muscle and joint pains persist then intermittent pain medication is required; if recurrent diverticulitis, constipation, or diarrhea exist they can be managed with medication; when too much stress is placed on the pumping action of a partly damaged heart, a metabolic blockade with cardiac medication is needed; and if blood pressure and blood sugar are outside normal ranges then they can be controlled with medication to ward off potentially serious consequences. Also, there are some specific medications that can enhance quality of life for those with cancer.

One significant issue in medical care that merits reconsideration is the use of drugs designed to prevent disease rather than trying to manage quality of life once disease has been identified. It is in this area that the greatest disagreement arises among physicians, pharmaceutical companies, and politicians.

The first issue to consider is whether preventive medicine has been responsible for expanding the number of elders in our population. This is partly true because people between 30 and 65 years of age, with specifically diagnosed diseases, have had an increase in survival by using drugs to correct glucose, lipid, and cholesterol levels; to reduce obesity; and to control hypertension. On the other hand, we counter with two points: 1) Access to cardiac, carotid artery, and aorta surgery; earlier diagnoses of cancer and improved surgical techniques for breast and prostate cancers; and successful campaigns against smoking and for the use of seatbelts have had a major effect on longevity that probably outweighs the effects of preventive drugs. 2) Even if the kinds of drugs described above have provided some protection to at-risk populations in the middle years of life, there is poor evidence that this protection continues into older ages past 70 years. We argue that ensuring that all members of the population, including elders, have rapid access to affordable diagnostic and surgical care to resolve potential life-threatening emergencies is the way to protect longevity—not years of daily medications.

A second issue in need of review is the use of heroic measures during the last months of one's life that are designed to prolong life for a brief time, but not necessarily to improve quality of life. As described throughout this book, heroic measures are responsible for the greatest part of each person's health care costs even though they do not appear to produce the desired benefits in significant addition of years of life or augmenting the quality of life. Measures like intensive chemotherapy for cancers that tend not to respond to treatment, such as lung, pancreas, and bowel cancers as well as longterm renal dialysis, major heart and lung surgery (including transplants), and intensive heart and lung maintenance procedures in intensive care units should only be considered after careful thought and a second medical opinion.

Occupying a hospital bed seems unnecessary and undesirable when needed attention can be given by health providers or family in one's own home. Although this may be challenging for some family members, clearly it is the humane and most cost-effective option when the end of life is near.

Unfortunately, many physicians are ill-prepared to present compassionate and palliative care options to their patients. As we discussed earlier, the role of the physician as comforter has been replaced by the medical bureaucracy's push to ensure that patients receive the most recent specialized technological care. Although many families have been reluctant to plan for the inevitable end of life, it appears that patients and their immediate families must decide what will make them most comfortable, and then take on the burden of instructing their health care provider as to their wishes (see chapter 6).

Issues Regarding Public Policy of Health Care

8

The Politics of Your Health Care

When we use the word "politics" we mean it in the most general sense of social decision-making, not just government action or inaction on issues. The biggest challenge we face is the necessity of careful planning for and after retirement to make certain we live out our lives in a state or a country that respects older members of the society. One thinks immediately of ancient societies where elders were respected and their advice sought, such as among the American Indians or in African or Asian village communities. But remember, we grew up during the second half of the 20th century in a society where Abbie Hoffman, a political and anti-war activist, intoned the now famous quotation, "Don't listen to anyone over 30!"

If it is not possible to achieve a reasonable level of respect where you live, you had better change the place where you live. (In the United States, the selection process is likely to become easier over time as it appears that each one of the 50 states will offer different levels of care and protection for those over 65.) When you identify a location that engenders reasonable respect for elders, you must then be sure that there are a number of other social-political components in place, including adequate pension payment systems, good health care programs, and adequate social support structures for your lifetime.

Many necessary political changes will occur only as the younger generation ages (that means that your author may miss out, but we can think of the wonderful prospects for our children and grandchildren!). For example, if one is indoctrinated at an early age to set aside a portion of income for health care and costs of living for that time when he or she no longer has a salary, there will be fewer financial challenges when age creeps into that person's life.

When young people apply for work, they should make it clear to potential employers that companies have an obligation to participate in pension plans or matching 401Ks as well as disability and health insurance if they expect to have satisfied, devoted employees. This approach will be considered by some as daydreaming, particularly in this time of economic recession. We argue that it is not. We believe a workforce that lacks human protective systems (including disability insurance and health care, pensions, and provisional allowance for maternity and family leave and disability) is a negative direction in social attitudes that has led and will continue to lead to a dysfunctional society.

Decades ago, unions were formed to protect workers against the prevailing agenda in place at the turn of the 20th century that allowed employers to establish subpar work standards that failed to provide workers with adequate wages, benefits, or safety measures solely to maximize profits. Many victories were achieved, including establishment of the minimum wage, workman's compensatory insurance (workers' comp), reasonable working hours, overtime compensation, etc., but there remains a long fight ahead as many of those achievements are being rolled back.

The conflict for social justice will soon move to the arena of health care for workers and retirees. The present method of taxing a shrinking workforce to maintain the current Medicare and Medicaid programs is already under attack for not being sound economic policy. As federal funds decrease, the federal deficit grows (and federal funds are less available), calls for higher taxes are shouted down, and public health care services shrink, a growing conflict is inevitable.

Some argue that health care and work safety should be a matter of personal choice, not a social mandate. We take the opposite view. This book is a tool to help those of you who believe in living as a member of society to foster a social conscience at an early age, to focus on human dignity and independence, to secure high quality health care, and to live without the threat of lost wages, waning pensions, inadequate housing, or absent health care.

In their book, *Taking Charge of Your Health*, Burton and Hall outlined the complexity and inefficiency of the Medicare system in the United States. They stated that the system is too complex, provides incomplete care, and is in urgent need of reform. Burton and Hall make a case for reform.

Indeed, health care has become very complex, incomplete, and is in urgent need of reform. We describe in the next two chapters just what those reforms might be and how only an assertive and unified voice will achieve better health care for the aging population.

Real change must start with an acceptance by the entire population that some sort of health insurance plan is essential. Two models for such plans are: 1) an income tax system that is adequate to cover all health care (as it exists in France, Canada, the United Kingdom, and Germany) and 2) a mandated health insurance plan with payments commencing at age 18 and covering all children in families (such as the model in Switzerland and in the state of Massachusetts).

At present, the voluntary system that exists in the United States cannot really be considered health insurance at all—rather, it is a selected health prepayment plan. Unless one participates in an employer-subsidized health plan, the voluntary system is predominantly for the wealthy because individual health insurance is impossibly expensive. Health insurance companies justify the high cost by arguing that those who buy health insurance do so because they anticipate illness in the near future or because they are older or already ill.

There is also a segment of the population in the United States that claims everyone should care for his or her self and, that by paying into an insurance system when they are healthy, they are being forced to pay for the health care of someone else. Although this may be true, spreading the risks and benefits of living together in a society is what humanity is all about.

Political leaders in most states agreed to pass legislation about 50 years ago that requires everyone who drives a car to have automobile insurance, regardless of their driving record. Therefore, those of us who drive carefully are constantly subsidizing careless drivers who tend to have accidents. Yet, required auto insurance has wide acceptance among drivers—perhaps because the need to drive is immediate and the penalties for not carrying insurance are very clear to everyone. But for some reason, the same individuals will not apply the same approach to health care insurance. It appears that a major social upheaval may be required before the idea of community-wide or nationwide protection is considered.

The United States Congress enacted the Social Security system on August 14, 1935, following the disastrous collapse of the financial system in 1929. In Europe, inclusive health care plans followed World War II when societal groups acknowledged that every individual was vulnerable to illness or injury. We hope such a massive upheaval will not be necessary before a majority of people in the United States start to think as a cohesive community. Although health care reform is being discussed in the United States, the danger of a meltdown in health care is ever present with no solution in sight.

This author provided direct medical care to patients for 30 years, spent over a decade designing drug trials for new medications, and spent many years in the university-based academic medical system in a department of public health. Departments of Public Health in universities and government settings emerged in the United States at the end of the 1800s in response to the need for communities to work together to solve large-scale problems like insect-related infectious diseases (malaria and yellow fever), waterborne diseases (typhoid, hepatitis, and polio), air pollution problems (respiratory illnesses), and the spread of contagious illnesses (influenza and tuberculosis). Better city sanitation and the creation and availability of vaccines to prevent communicable diseases were milestones in public health. Each of these programs required significant financial cost at every level of the social network (town, county, state, federal), but mostly they required a concept of social or public participation. This demonstrated a sharp difference in thinking from the popular Wild West (frontier) free-spirit, personal-risk, and personal-gain mentality that could not solve these immense problems. Over the past 200 years, people living in the United States have come to accept community police forces, fire departments, public school systems, insect control programs, water purification, and vaccination programs but not adequate health care and reasonable pension plans.

Vaccination programs have been limited in Switzerland where certain groups (mainly naturalists and anthroposophists) have concluded and widely advertised their opinion that vaccination is a matter of individual freedom and personal choice rather than public health. As a result, Switzerland is experiencing a measles epidemic long after the disease has been controlled in most of the world—next, we expect, will be a recurrence of polio, pertussis, and diphtheria! The Swiss children now suffering (and dying) from measles, of course, had no voice in these decisions.

As recently as 50 years ago in the United States, city and county hospitals would take care of all ill people arriving at their doors, but not anymore. Now one needs cash or an insurance card to get anything other than emergency medical care and, even then, the cost of the care is unknown until long after the patient has survived or died. The lack of complete health care insurance for all its people has put the United States low on the list of a humanity index for its communities. The United States ranks 41 among nations of the world for life expectancy. Few private-practice physicians accept Medicaid patients and a growing number of physicians will not accept a new patient if they are on Medicare—the justification being too many complex forms to complete and too little reimbursement to support the time of the physician and staff. Patients in search of a general practitioner have fewer and fewer options.

As we know, the United States based its existence on the concept ". . . of the people, by the people, and for the people. . . ." This is troubling in view of the fact that a majority of people in the United States do not seem to want a universal health care system. As difficult as this is to believe, it appears to be a fact. So how can one propose a system that has been proven to work in many countries if the people of the United States do not want it? First, read chapter 11, which describes how lawmakers are thinking about solving the problem. And here we recommend some social and political actions that can be carried out immediately—they require only thought and action.

1. **Work with local advocacy groups** to try to establish a combination of payment plans that will cover all expenses for prescription medications, medical care, and hospitalization for those 65 years of age or older. If reasonable health care is to continue, the system must be adjusted to require that those over 65 have private comprehensive health insurance and/or that a federal or state system of taxes is in place to ensure that supplemental insurance is available for complete coverage. To make the system viable, younger Americans will have to purchase lifetime health care insurance and contribute a greater percentage of their salaries to county, state, and federal taxes specifically for health care.

These changes will have to be regulated in some way by a local oversight board. At present, a very small percentage of the population carry longterm health care insurance for several reasons: first, the cost is prohibitive; second, many Americans believe that their taxes designated for health care are already too high and should provide for that need; and third, people believe themselves to be immortal.

We estimate that if health care insurance becomes more widely available at a reasonable cost, approximately 65% of the population will acquire appropriate coverage through health care plans provided, in part, by employers and partly from personal funds; and approximately 35% will require county, state, or federal tax dollars to ensure their coverage, or a combination of both personal and government subsidies. If appropriate health care is put in place for all, then the system should be adequately funded for those over 65. It will take years to work out the details of this plan and it will place a heavy burden on young people and the companies they work for to do the necessary social planning that determines the kind of coverage they want (the private insurance component is described in detail in a subsequent chapter) and what kind of coverage they would rather have covered by taxes.

2. **Help establish a health care watchdog and information agency** to ensure that information being provided to physicians regarding medication guidelines is accurate and appropriate, and that there is a specific focus on real quality of life issues for patients rather than simply a chart of statistics. At present, physicians are not given the tools and support systems necessary to deal with the overwhelming amount of data from pharmaceutical companies and medical associations that promote and prescribe prescription drugs. This agency would also monitor the use, or overuse, of laboratory tests and extraordinary and very costly procedures like MRIs. An important role for a "watchdog" agency would be to ensure that the pharmaceutical industry's direct-to-patient advertising be appropriate and truthful. Years ago, cigarette ads were banned from television because cigarettes were considered a significant health risk to the population. At some point, we hope that same consideration will be given to prescription drug ads that have greatly increased drug consumption and have contributed to the explosion in health care costs.

3. **Search out in advance the services you may need in the future,** including in-home care services, longterm rehabilitation or nursing facilities, physical activity and day care centers for partly disabled or Alzheimer's patients, and rapid hospital or emergency

facilities. These are difficult things to think about when you are vital and well, but advanced preparation is essential to ensure adequate care and also to be certain you receive exactly the care and support you want—not what others may choose for you when you are not able to choose for yourself.

Find and utilize adult gyms that include cardio equipment and groups that enjoy swimming, water aerobics, bicycling, jogging, or walking excursions. Many of these should be included as part of Medicare insurance and/or be supported by local taxes in your community, like public pools and tennis or handball courts.

9

Examples of Health Care Insurance Plans and Government Health Care Taxation Approaches

Here we describe health care insurance developed in Switzerland to demonstrate how all citizens can have full health care coverage, the approach in Canada to provide coverage to all citizens via government taxation, the health care plan developed in several states in the United States, and the Affordable Care Act established by the current administration and scheduled to go into effect in 2013. No one system is perfect, and each one needs timely review and revision as the population ages and health care expenses increase. Some form of regulation and oversight, probably by a legislative body, will be required to assess the efficiency and adequacy of any system and to propose changes as necessary.

In Switzerland, the healthcare system was designed to be a fully private health insurance plan. The role of the Swiss government is to regulate the process by: 1) requiring each person over the age of 18 years, and following the completion of their education, to obtain the insurance (that also includes coverage for all of the children of insured individuals); and 2) providing oversight and supervision of the more than 80 health care insurance companies that offer health insurance plans.

There are two potential flaws in the Swiss system: first is the constant concern that there be a level playing field for all of the insurance companies—fairness and transparency are essential. Companies that offer less expensive premium plans may be excluding elders or those with known diseases and may be focusing instead on the young and healthy who require less costly services. The problem is that as one ages or acquires some disease risk, the inexpensive plans do not provide the best service and when individual policy holders attempt to change companies, it becomes either very expensive or impossible. Although there are rather strict rules Swiss insurance companies must follow, the process of changing insurance policies and the steep cost involved requires constant oversight. In contrast, in the United States there are rules specifically prohibiting "cherry picking" (assigning a person to a particular plan based on their good health; i.e., the person's low cost/high profit to the insurance company), though subtle ways to circumvent the rules are still in place and may be difficult to detect.

The second potential flaw in the Swiss system is the lack of intervention by the insurance companies or the government regulators to control costs of pharmaceuticals and new technology. The cost of a physician's consultation time and in-hospital duration are controlled, but these make up only a small part of the total health care cost. Health care has become more and more expensive, as it has everywhere, but there appears to be insufficient attention to why the costs are rising or how costs can be controlled. If the government were to intervene excessively, despite such intervention being needed, Swiss citizens who pride themselves on private health care formulas would complain bitterly about government intervention in an otherwise successful business arrangement.

As a result of this partial hands-off approach to cost containment, health care costs in Switzerland appear high compared to health care costs in other countries. This is made more difficult to calculate because the cost of everything in Switzerland is higher than elsewhere, as are wages and benefits. Rather than discuss the exchange rates of Swiss francs to other currencies, it looks like the best comparison is by the so-called McDonald hamburger exchange rate. This rate currently makes a Big Mac more than twice as expensive in Switzerland as in the United States (actually the cost of such a hamburger in Switzerland is the highest in the world).

Most Swiss people are happy to keep the health care system as it is but the need for insurance company regulation and federal supervision of health care costs remain ever present in the background. Most individuals pay 5% to 10% o f their income toward insurance. This is not tax deductible since it is considered a part of the social welfare system, just as are the taxes that pay for education (including university) and all the usual taxes for personal safety (fire, police, sanitation, and military), road construction, and government operations. If someone's health care insurance premium exceeds 10% of their income, government revenue (at least in some of the 26 cantons in Switzerland) can be used to pay the difference between the 10% and the amount charged by the insurance company.

Within the context of careful government oversight, the Swiss health insurance companies have done a reasonably good job of calculating how those at high risk pay a few percentage points more for their health insurance than those at low risk. It is important to note that the individual being insured chooses the insurance company, not the reverse. Therefore, the problem of "cherry picking" only occurs when an insured person decides that he or she needs better coverage. Then, when he or she attempts to change companies, he or she can be refused or there can be restrictions pertaining to previous illnesses. Thus, a young healthy person is faced with a gamble but, in general, the moderately priced to more expensive plans are selected because people are aware of these problems and their potential future consequences.

The Swiss system includes several obvious mechanisms: 1) If the individual being insured has never had a health problem, they may get a rebate of 15% of the cost. 2) If the insured person starts to have medical problems, there is a mechanism for the insurance company to increase his or her premium, though the increase is relatively small compared to the overall cost of insurance premiums for health care and seldom exceeds a few percentage points of annual income. 3) Individuals can choose the amount they pay each year—with a less expensive policy, there will be higher self-pay amounts before the insurance begins and/or fewer deductibles. 4) Corporations contribute to the insurance coverage of their employees (often about 15%) and this gives a sort of collective bargaining position for those being insured. 5) If and/or when a Swiss resident is unable to pay for insurance, then he or she applies to the appropriate office (unemployment, immigration, pensions, etc.) and the government tax payments come into effect to ensure continued coverage. The main point to remember is that health insurance is a legal requirement, not an option, for all residents. The Swiss example is one method of financing health care delivery. Several other European countries have a mixed system of privately purchased insurance and government payment via taxation.

Now let us look at the system that imposes a federal tax to provide health care to ensure complete health care coverage for all citizens.

The best example is the National Health Service (NHS) in the United Kingdom, where providers and health care institutions are part of the government structure and all citizens are assigned primary care providers that are financed by national taxes. Resources are allocated to regional health councils based on the number of people in the region, and decisions on how resources are spent are made jointly based on national guidelines and local directives.

As we were growing up in the 1950s, we were taught that any form of "socialized medicine" was one of the worst things that a country could contemplate, let alone implement. The main target of criticism was the United Kingdom, but France and a few other countries were included. The generally accepted idea then was that socialized medicine meant no choice of physician, no choice of specialist referrals, underpaid and angry medical care workers, and especially that the chronically ill were benefiting at the expense of the well (who, it was assumed, could attribute their good health to their good lifestyle). The concept also suggested bureaucratic inefficiency and dispersal of funds in directions other than to the care of patients. Health care in the United States, at that time, was considered a privilege not a right.

We who listened to these criticisms 50 years ago must now accept that we were misinformed. It is now clear that a much higher percentage of citizens of the UK, France, and Germany have an opportunity for complete health care than do citizens in the United States. In addition, physicians in these countries are content with acting as care providers rather than small business proprietors. The problems of cost containment remain but as the UK debates whether to partially privatize their system, it is interesting to watch and listen to outcries from the citizens insisting that new laws not permit even small parts of their health care system to be thrown away.

The citizens do not want to risk damage to an excellent program to satisfy misguided attempts to solve problems during an economic recession caused by factors completely unrelated to the health care bureaucracy. It is of special note that Finland, Sweden, and Denmark have health care from birth to death funded entirely by tax revenue, and absolutely no one is suggesting that those systems be altered.

There are less odious forms of national health care that people in the United States can examine. Here we describe the Canadian system in 2012. The system in Canada was derived from the concepts in England and France, but it is chosen as an example because Canada resembles the United States in so many ways both historically and geographically. It is important to note that there is no single National Health Plan in Canada. The plan is composed of interlocking territorial plans (13 territories and provinces) that share the principles described by the federal government in what is called the Canadian Health Act.

This act describes a system in which the costs are financed by general tax revenues, with each region receiving a global capped budget as well as guidelines for use of territorial resources.

The first step in the Canadian plan is primary health care that is publicly funded by general tax revenues. Once a referral to a specialized hospital or longterm care facility has been made, provincial and territorial governments pay the cost. Patients may pay for room and board in a longterm health care facility but all shortterm hospital or nursing care is covered by tax revenue. Individual services, such as vision care, dental care, prescriptions outside of the hospital, and services of allied health providers, vary across Canada and are sometimes, but not always, covered by supplementary private insurance plans. Territories and provinces provide coverage for alternative health care of various types, and always include coverage of certain groups including elders and children. Under the Canadian Health Act, all drugs administered in hospitals are publicly funded but outside of the hospital, the territorial governments are responsible and the level of coverage may vary. As a result, most Canadians take advantage of coverage through either private or publicly funded prescription drug programs.

In summary, this program of national health care is complex, but universal, and attempts to ensure that all Canadians have the health care they need provided by a combination of federal, provincial, and territorial tax funding, supplemented by private insurances, particularly for medications used outside of the hospital setting.

Let us now turn to the complex issue of how various states in the United States have chosen to deal with health care coverage. We will also examine several specific counties, as it used to be a tradition in the United States that health care was a county responsibility (as noted by the functioning of county hospitals, the regulation of physician activities by county medical societies, and the provision of care to the poorest by county social care boards), and was funded in a large part via property taxes (the main source of funding for county activities). The United States is a fascinating example of diversity in many ways and the methods of health care are no exception. It must be of some comfort for elders in the United States to know they need not leave the country in order to have some security regarding their health care and its financing. We have chosen several states to demonstrate the diversity of plans currently available.

The state of Massachusetts has been very much in the news recently regarding its health care plan. In 2006, Massachusetts enacted the Healthcare Insurance Reform Law that required all state residents to carry a minimum level of health insurance coverage or to be eligible for government health care insurance contingent on low levels of income. The result of this legislation is a health care plan similar to that of Switzerland's with the exception that a greater percentage of people depend on the government-paid insurance than in Switzerland.

Recent numbers show that, in Massachusetts, 16.4% of residents are covered by Medicare, 16.6% by public plans like Commonwealth Care and Medicaid, and 65.1% by employer-subsidized group insurance coverage. This results in over 98% of Massachusetts residents having health care payment security (the highest in the nation). The remaining 2% are able to prove they have no access to affordable insurance or they cannot participate for religious reasons (these residents must pay a tax penalty for not being insured).

There are ongoing challenges to the Massachusetts system, including the fact that health care costs have not been reduced by the plan, and there are currently legal challenges to various sections of the law. Neither of these challenges were unexpected since the plan did not target methods to reduce the rising costs of health care, nor would one expect such a broad-based plan to be implemented without legal questions being raised. In an earlier chapter we examined how these insurance plans cover other aspects of care for elders, such as nursing care, rehabilitation, in-home care, and nursing home payments.

California is another state with a history of strong state government support of health care. This has changed rather dramatically over several decades and it is still in the process of revision, but it remains a valuable example of health care in the United States. In California, an attempt is being made to initiate a comprehensive health care plan (designated as *State Bill (SB) 810*). If passed, the bill would establish a universal plan paid for by state taxes, rather than by individual private health care insurance.

This plan is similar to the plans in the United Kingdom and in Canada, and is entirely different from the Massachusetts plan. The pending bill is entitled *Health Care for All* and has recently passed the California State Health Committee.

California's so-called *Single Payer Bill* was approved twice by the state legislature (2006 and 2008) but was vetoed both times by, then Governor, Arnold Schwarzenegger. At present, it is awaiting reconsideration by the current state legislature. It is particularly interesting that this bill represents an attempt to reduce administrative costs and control rising costs for health care, while at the same time providing medical health care to all California residents. Critics of the proposed California plan have stated it is so comprehensive that, if enacted, people would flock to California just to take advantage of its complete health care system. To prevent that from happening, there might be a minimum duration of residency requirement included in the law.

The examples of health care in Massachusetts and California demonstrate how complete health care can be provided by two completely different systems (private insurance or government taxation). We have examples of other states where health care is either partially or completely avoided by state or county funding mechanisms. To provide this information, your authors went to several state internet websites.

After fairly exhaustive searches, it is clear that detailed information services are available in both Ohio and Alaska, but the only real health care plans are actually state administered Medicare and Medicaid programs. Due to the uncertain financial status of Medicare and Medicaid, it is likely that these two states' health plans are uncertain as well. In Oregon, there is a mix of health care insurances. In the executive summary of Oregon's insurance plan, it is recorded that 39% of residents have insurance from commercial insurers, 26% have Medicare of Medicaid, 18% have employer-based coverage, and 17% (617,000 residents) are uninsured. After reviewing information from a number of states, it seems to us that no state has a solution to the impending federal health care crisis except, possibly, California and Massachusetts.

Another major health care issue requires careful consideration. For the past 20 years in the United States, health care planners and providers have grappled with serious flaws in the health care system that has increasingly leaned toward what is now known as "managed care." The concept of managed care came into sharp focus after the United States Congress rejected plans by the Clinton administration to revise national health care funding. Instead, in 1994, the United States Congress, backed by private investors, insurance companies, and a few health care organizations, chose a privately funded mechanism in an attempt to reduce health care costs and redistribute health care availability. We believed then that the choice to opt for a managed care system was the wrong choice. Now, it is apparent to almost everyone that this approach has been a disastrous failure for all, not just for those over 65.

The process of managing health care in the United States would be fascinating to watch if the managed care experiment had not become so destructive to patient care, physician practices, and to financial investors. In view of the current uncertainties of the socio-economic landscape within the United States and internationally, it is difficult to predict what the ultimate outcome will be. How is it that people with reasonable intellect in a democratic, ethically based, health care-conscious society never created a stable equitable health care system for all of their citizens?

Most of us grew up in the United States when doctors provided medical care as either general practitioners or specialists. There was a perception among many that physicians were being too well paid and that this led to a problem in access to health care. Although few physicians we knew were examples of an economic windfall, we believe that the system was not very efficient.

Years ago, physician work hours were long, there were frequent house calls, academic research projects were carried out while also taking care of a full roster of patients, and making morning rounds and teaching medical students and resident physicians were all part of the expectations for doctors in academic medicine.

The system could have been improved if medical planners and health care bureaucrats had observed the system and anticipated its breakdown. That was not done. Instead, managed care was put in place as an experiment in financial restructuring. Managed care emerged without a thought of establishing ethical standards in the delivery of health care to replace traditional standards. Managed care allowed a system of commercialism to substitute for the physician's guardian role in health care. One result of a top-heavy bureaucratic management structure has been escalating costs that have left many people without access to health care at all. Physicians are now trying to rebalance their humanitarianism, their medical ethics, their independence, their very existence within this system, but years of restructuring the once functional, albeit inefficient, system has made a major correction seem nearly impossible.

How did it happen that health care—once a traditionally humanitarian process with its core rooted in the doctor-patient relationship, with its demanding educational requirements, with its social focus at the edge of all aspects of birth, life, fear, pain and death—became a primarily commercial activity? We can point out a few key elements that may have led to the present managed care industry in the United States.

In many ways, managed care is a product of the technological revolution. Two major issues have resulted from the infusion of new technology into medical care. 1) The expectations created by new technology and the resulting expense in dollars has led to a tremendous gap between patient demands and the funds available for health care delivery. New technology created the demand and then the economic sector, not the medical-ethical sector, was tapped to solve the problem. 2) In the past those that practiced medicine provided comfort and support to their patients, partly because there was no special technology available to intervene in the illness of their patients. We must ask the question, therefore, how can we provide the most up-to-date technology to each patient without losing the humanitarian component provided by the physician? In other words, the question is whether technology and humanity are mutually exclusive. The answer is, "No."

Physicians must be taught how to evaluate the appropriate technology for each patient (that is to apply ethical considerations, not economic ones), and then they must learn how to refer each patient, in the most thoughtful way, to those who can deliver the new technology (that is to be a wise comforter). Both activities must be done efficiently and must utilize processes learned during medical education—these are not merely management skills. We must then have a system to ensure that the physician is appropriately reimbursed for his actions at each level of a patient's care. This is a civil-social process, not a management process. It is our opinion that the way new technology would affect patient care was never considered at the start of this revolution. Indeed, what happened was that patients saw their physicians become more and more distant;

there was ever-greater attention given to tests and computerized documentation and less attention to human interaction, which resulted in a new breed of "primary care physician" (the PCP) replacing the trusted family doctor. Financial cost to the patient increased dramatically, humane treatment decreased, and, finally, the process evolved into a purely commercial managed system.

In retrospect, underestimating the financial cost of new technology and its resulting impact on the system was not the only mistake made in the 1970s, but perhaps the biggest mistake was installing a bureaucratic referral system between a patient and a specialist that often requires batteries of expensive tests and procedures to justify the referral. This led us all in the wrong direction—toward non-medical bureaucracy and commercialism, rather than toward expert physician-directed humanitarian use of new technology. We should never have permitted the creation of an entirely non-medical access layer.

One dream of those supporting managed health care was that by adding efficient management the poor distribution of health care in the United States would be solved. On the surface, this thinking seemed reasonable because technology was thought to be far too complex for a mere patient and physician to sort out. It was thought that if health care was not available to all, it was most likely the result of an inefficient delivery system.

In the present managed care environment, the poor distribution of care persists but the economics of the system puts money into different pockets. The message is clear—poor distribution of health care cannot be remedied by bringing in market-driven administrators and economists; better health care can only be achieved by designing a system that distributes health care dollars in a manner that ensures the availability of preventive medical care, good nutrition, and, when needed, medical intervention to all. This would, by necessity, be a very large industry combining taxation, insurance, and efficient decision-making—perhaps as large as the present defense industry—and why not?

In the plan we envision, the physician would be the comforter, the technologist, the ethicist, and the provider in the system. Health care planners and politicians would have to be involved in establishing the infrastructure but the system goal would be a humanitarian health care solution, not financial gain for a few. The absence of a humane goal is the major failure of the managed care experiment in the United States.

One reason the managed care experiment was done in the United States and not elsewhere was the American enthusiasm for the marketplace as a social balance. An underlying current of opinion suggested that good people deserve things but do not require a support system, whereas bad people do not deserve things and they do require a costly support system; so market forces would level the imbalances in the system. The movement toward managed care in the United States will be discussed for a long time but our belief is that the real benefit of the experiment will be to point out the fallacy in the direction taken. Market forces will never set as a goal the kind of humanitarian activities needed to ensure the health care of a society. Market forces are not likely able to save the market, let alone the well-being of individuals in a society.

One must ask where the medical leadership was during this process. The American Medical Association (AMA) has guided medical practice in the United States for a long time. This organization is the principal physicians' organization in the United States and has done many good things. The AMA has served as a major source of information exchange; they have been a bridge between physician care and political/legal/para-physician organizations; and, most of all, they have been a force to promote the established system of providing health care. Regrettably, at a critical time in the medical restructuring process of the 1980s, the AMA failed to provide the needed perspective as the guardian of health. This was due, in part, to cultural fears that led to the rejection of the Clinton Administration's proposal for sweeping new health care reforms, but also because of the AMA's traditional role as a physicians' union.

It is true that the ethical issues related to new plans for a health care system were discussed, but recommendations arising from these discussions were placed on the back burner. Had the AMA acknowledged the problems of access to health care, distribution of fees, inadequate attention to preventive health care, and lack of clarity and consistency in hospital admissions and the use of new technologies, it might have been in a better position as a respected organization to contribute to the solution. More recently, spokesmen within the AMA have tried to alter the course of events. The American College of Physicians has called on all physicians to become leaders in the movement to achieve universal access to health care but, by all appearances, these activities are too little too late.

Now there is a more dangerous aspect to the managed care apparatus. It is a growing trend for health insurance companies in the United States to invest in HMOs—they collect patients' money, use part of it to pay the health care bill (after the patient has paid a co-pay or deductible amount), then they receive the money back as an investor. This is a clever financial arrangement but it is not health care. The cost of health care is not decreasing—instead, we see an increasing amount of money going to CEOs and corporate managers and investors rather than to the structure and delivery of quality health care.

The message here is that physicians and physician organizations must be at the forefront of innovative efforts to solve social-medical problems, rather than serving as the primary vehicle for preserving the status quo. Changing the scenario will be no easy task since a major role for most physician-derived organizations is to protect the financial status of its members.

If we look at what has happened to health care in the United States and consider what is likely to occur in the next year or so, we can expect a heightened stimulus to identify the form of any innovative health care plan. Until recently, no one envisioned that part of the medical care meltdown in the United States would be the bankruptcy of physicians caused by serious financial mistakes made by the managed care facilities they work for. The good news about managed health care organizations is that we can learn from their mistakes; we can also take advantage of the efficiency and success achieved by some of them, like Kaiser Permanente in California or Health Partners in Minnesota.

10

Medicare and Medicaid Health Plans—Designed to Fail?

This chapter is written with a great sense of frustration and disappointment. When the Medicare plan was first adopted by Congress and signed into law by President Lyndon Johnson in 1964, we all believed that a new era of social responsibility had emerged in the United States. Sadly, due primarily to inadequate funding and absent regulatory supervision, we have learned that the plan was destined to fail from the beginning. We now know that the economic planners involved in Medicare creation were na ve to believe that a health care system designed to benefit those over 65 could survive in a country that: votes against new general obligation taxes, favors the private sector vs. government action as a fulfillment mechanism, is willing to accumulate vast amounts of private debt (via high-interest-rate credit cards) but will not increase taxes by a single penny to pay for health care, and believes that youth is eternal.

A more cynical explanation for the Medicare plan is that the economic planners who created it were swayed by investment bankers holding excess cash that they wanted to turn into profit by having a guaranteed, high-quality debtor—the United States Federal Government. They envisioned that everyone would be happy—the government would have a health plan that would appear to cost tax payers very little by adding only a little more in employment taxes, and the financial institutions would have a reliable income. Everyone was happy until the mortgage and housing markets collapsed in 2009 and United States credit reached a ceiling in 2011—payback time had arrived.

From the beginning of the Medicare program, each person paying the health employment tax used about three times the amount put in after he or she began receiving health care after age 65. Richard Nixon and Edward Kennedy tried to reform the Medicare and Medicaid laws in 1974, and then the Clinton administration tried in the 1990s, but Congress did not approve any of the reforms. Then, during the Bush administration, taxes were reduced for the wealthiest Americans and the United States entered two new wars, making it impossible to pay for health care. Health care tax revenue was less than $200 billion per year, but health care costs to the federal government were over $500 billion annually. The dilemma was best described in an Associated Press article that explained how a married couple would have to pay an average $114,000 in health care-designated employment taxes during their working years, but their medical expenses after age 65 would be $353,000—300% more than what they paid in. Thus, the cost of Medicare was not even covered for those who paid, let alone by the 33% of American society that did not pay employment tax.

We now know that Medicare and Medicaid have survived for the past few decades but Federal taxes have not paid for them—rather, the money has been borrowed from China, the Arab countries, Europe, and world and U.S. banking consortiums. What a plan— offer complete health care to elders then just borrow the money to pay for it.But how does the debt get paid back?

Let us explore the problems that have accumulated in the Medicare and Medicaid plans and then suggest a few options to get out of the mess. The biggest problem was faulty logic in the original plan—the idea that one could pay 3% of his or her income via an employment tax while under 65 years old and still working, but would not pay the amount needed beyond age 65. It is true that social security payments are taxed, but that revenue is not targeted for health care. The idea of absent payment for health care after age 65 completely negated several important facts.

First, the cost of the program and resources to fund it were underestimated: a) People over 65 have largely stopped making many of the expenditures necessary when they were younger (like for college tuition and home mortgages), therefore they would have more financial flexibility to pay for health care than they did when they were younger; b) Increasing health care payments by those already retired, from 3%, to 10%, to 15% of their pension income, would be necessary to provide relief for the working young who have heavy payment burdens; c) There are many people over 65 who have ample capacity to pay for their health care because of pensions and investment plans—so why should the government go into debt to provide such funds? The best example of this was the issuance of the first two Medicare cards to Harry and Bess Truman—two people certainly able to pay for their health care in full.

A second problem was the failure to install an adequate regulatory system to monitor payments via Medicare and Medicaid. The government has the resources to audit only about 5% of all annual payments, thus leaving the door open to fraud and corruption that has cost billions in misappropriated funds with no hope of recouping them. The level of fraud in the Medicare and Medicaid systems is particularly disturbing since much of it is done by health care professionals who have the responsibility of taking care of their patients rather than ripping off the system. To read that a governor of Florida cannot stop major prescription fraud in his state because he does not have the resources to prosecute the fraudsters should cause outrage among the citizenry and Congress. Even more astonishing, one fraudster on being discovered fled to Cuba! Regulation should be the first step in organizing any federal or state program, not the last step.

The third problem is that there appears to be little interest or willingness to control the increasing costs of health care. The only present effort is to put a cap on the amount of payments to physicians and hospital in-patient services. This has led to an increase in physicians refusing to accept Medicare patients, and hospitals limiting in-patient stays. Examining the causes of increased costs appears to be totally ignored. This subject was discussed in chapter 6.

The concept that because we are living longer we need more financing of ever more health care is likely wrong but remains untested. One can argue (and it has been reported) that most major health events occur at the end of life (most commonly due to cancer, vascular disease, or pulmonary insufficiency) but do not occur each year between age 65 and the time of death. Many of the annual costs may well be due to the inappropriate use of medications, diagnostic tests, and procedures, but the major cost is ineffective heroic end-of-life treatments. Each aging person should be aggressive in examining this issue in his or her own life. After careful consideration, we must each make the choice to purchase catastrophic illness or medi-gap insurance; discuss with our medical care provider what is really vital in our daily regimen; reject all of the direct advertising in magazines and on television about the latest wonder treatments; and then place our Medicare cards in a drawer and go about being the healthy young people hidden within each of us.

When we come to the politics of a federal health care system, one can see that citizens of the United States are truly divided. The party lines are fairly clear, but the overall objective of each of the main parties is a bit confused. For example, on the right of the political spectrum one sees a desire for such limited government and taxation that one wonders how society could exist at all; the argument appears to be that the family should bear all burdens of an aging or ill parent while meeting their other financial obligations at the same time; or grandma and grandpa should just die and leave the family to go about the business of being young. On the left side of the spectrum, it appears that taxation should be an expected cost of running society, so pay up and keep on keeping on. At present, the United States population has chosen the path of least resistance—to pay for whatever is requested (multiple foreign wars, a big government bureaucracy, and lots of health care) by borrowing the money and paying 42 cents of every tax dollar to service the interest on the debt!

Another quandary that occupies the room when discussing the shambles of our Medicare and Medicaid programs is the immediate question, "What is the alternative?" We have discussed the facts that other countries have taken different routes and have been much more successful than the United States has been. That does not mean that the methods used in other countries could be applied now in the United States, with the exception, perhaps, of a modified Canadian system. The Swiss system would not be possible because the fraudulent behavior of health insurance companies might actually exceed that which is already occurring in the Medicare system. One need only talk to friends or relatives about how their insurance claims have been refused, or read *The Rainmaker*—John Grisham's novel about a young boy with leukemia who dies while his mother and her lawyer fight to hold their insurance company responsible for denying a claim for needed treatment—to understand that putting a system in place that empowers insurance companies to determine the health care of the nation would require major regulatory oversight of the insurance industry.

One insurance provider refused to reimburse a friend of this author's after she was admitted, unconscious, to a local hospital. Why? Because she did not sign the appropriate forms required to initiate insurance coverage—because?—she was unconscious!

In addition, there would have to be more competition among a much larger selection of plans. In Switzerland, the system works because there are more than 80 different companies each offering different plans—and all of the companies are carefully regulated. None would dare to refuse a legitimate claim presented by one of their clients for fear of losing their accreditation. It is clear that, in the United States, insurance companies act more like banks or holding companies designed to collect as much money as possible, pay out as little as possible, and then invest their cash reserves for the benefit of the corporate stock holders. This system would have to be changed if the nation were to rely solely on health insurance companies for its health care.

Our recommendations are as follows: 1) If federal, state, county, or city funds are to be used, all citizens must be included as recipients of health care—not just those over 65 or the impoverished or disabled. 2) If insurance companies are to be in the middle of health care, then there must be a diversity of plans, competition, and transparency. 3) If there is a combination of the two, there must be an organization responsible for oversight and regulation (checking 5% of federal payments or occasional legal proceedings against insurance companies is simply not good enough).

Here, and in the next chapter, are a few suggestions from the authors of this book, who are neither economists nor politicians but elders who deserve to have their voices heard. As the citizens of the United States endure a period of debt crisis (created by an economic plan approved by both republican and democratic congresses and administrations that placed borrowing as a lead part of social advancement), they appear unwilling to solve the discrepancy between income and payments.

One author of this book confronted his daughter about her willingness to continuously increase her debt and pay huge amounts in interest to credit card companies. Her answer was, as always, right on target: "Dad, you don't understand—it's the American way." So, our first suggestion is to somehow change the culture of the nation from spend now, pay later, to let us spend within our means. Of course, such a change appears impossible because it is cultural not logical, and partly because the loan industry would collapse, and because consumer inactivity would lead to increased unemployment and a true depression. In essence, every credit-overdrawn household would be participating in overthrowing the government they ultimately need to blame for the situation.

We also suggest: 1) Each person, starting at age 50, should put aside 5% to 10% of their income for future health care, and 15% for pension investments (that leaves 25% for taxes, and 50% for all other necessities of life). Even though income will decrease after age 65, the amount of 5% to 10% should remain. 2) As Medicare and Medicaid shrink or fail as a result of the need to pay off the national debt while not increasing taxes, we suggest that the Medicare components designated parts B, C, and D be continued as they are mainly funded by local governments, insurance, or out-of-pocket payments. Part A, payment to hospitals, must be severely diminished. The only way to deal with this shortfall will be to ask hospitals to downsize their services to be in line with their income—revenues can be increased somewhat by increasing costs to self-pay patients and insurance companies. Waste, corruption, unnecessary tests, and the astronomical costs of heroic treatments will have to be addressed. In addition, the cost of training resident physicians has to be revisited. Physician training used to be underwritten by the government, including the overhead costs of the training facilities. This reimbursement system was drastically changed about 20 years ago and those dollars cut. If we want to be a country that supports well-trained physicians and quality health care, we have to think seriously about how many of our tax dollars should be allocated to those costs. When hospitals return to the business of training physicians and caring for patients, rather than hiring CEOs (with their respective army of COOs, VPs, and SVPs—none of whom deliver one moment of health care) to operate hospitals as holding companies for ambulance companies and medical appliance catalogue companies, we might see an end to ever-rising health care costs.

The other option is to go to a system of community-based clinics with less access to tests and treatments currently provided by centralized hospitals. 3) We who are over 65 must do our part to demand that any medications, diagnostic procedures, and hospitalizations are essential to our quality of life. Many prescriptions and treatments have been sold to us as a means of extending our lives when what we really want is quality of life—financial security for the remaining period of our life, mobility, freedom from isolation, reasonable pain relief, and certainty that when the end of life comes, we will be in our own home or, for a reasonably short time, in a well-staffed hospital or hospice.

In the past 18 months, there has been no shortage of proposals, suggestions, and recommendations for controlling health care costs. A lot has been said about what needs to be accomplished but little is convincing in specifics. This is not the first time that voices within the federal government have realized that the United States needs major health care reform.

The proposals from the Nixon administration and later the Clinton administration never made it into law. In March, 2010, President Barack Obama signed the Federal Affordable Care Act that is to be fully implemented in 2013. This legislation was designed to improve health care throughout the nation and each state must participate in some manner. At present, the new plan is the subject of an on-going nationwide debate. It appears likely that this plan will never be fully implemented for a number of reasons—some fact-based, some not.

During 2012, other plans will likely be presented that do not have any chance of being enacted into law mostly because a significant group in the United States Congress is not willing to allocate the taxes that any reasonable program would require. Some of the proposals include converting Medicare from a fee-for-service program to a voucher/premium-support plan (linked to a nationwide private insurance exchange). The variations of these plans are discussed in chapter 11.

We all know the present system of health care in the United States is not working. We can work together to find alternatives using the same creative spirit that has been a part of this country since it was created. The sooner we start, the better.

11

Recent Proposals to Reform Medicare

That Medicare has cost problems is no secret. A brief review of the Trustees Report for 2011 is instructive. Total benefit expenditures for all of Medicare in 2010 were $515 billion, amounting to slightly less than $11,000 per beneficiary. According to the Report's intermediate projection, the number of beneficiaries will increase from 47.5 million in 2010 to nearly 64 million in 2020, with costs per beneficiary to grow to about $14,000. Note: the Trustees report admits that this projection is unrealistic, as it assumes Congress will permit the physician's payment rates to be reduced (by 29%) as stated in present law. This is unlikely to happen and, consequently, per beneficiary costs more realistically would reach $15,000 in 2020, a growth of more than 3% per year. Beyond that, there is no real relief in sight. The potential causes are many and complex (medical treatment practices, fear of liability, costs of technology, increasing average ages of the population, over-promotion of pharmaceuticals, insufficiently controlled fraudulent practices). Each health care constituency has its preference, but the answer is probably: All of the above.

Where can a solution be found? A quote from the Kaiser Family Foundation Focus on Health Care Reform (including Parts A and B premiums) summarizing the Patient Protection and Affordable

Care Act (so-called "Obama Care") highlights the difficulty of the problem. The act will establish an independent payment advisory board comprised of 15 members to submit legislative proposals containing recommendations to reduce the per capita rate of growth in Medicare spending if spending exceeds a target growth rate. Beginning April 2013, the act requires the chief actuary of CMS to project whether Medicare per capita spending exceeds the average of CPI-U and CPI-M, based on a five-year period ending that year. If so, beginning January 15, 2014, the board will submit recommendations to achieve reductions in Medicare spending.

Beginning January 2018, the target is modified such that the board submits recommendations if Medicare per capita spending exceeds GDP per capita plus one percent. The board will submit proposals to the president and Congress for immediate consideration. The board is prohibited from submitting proposals that would ration care; increase revenues; change benefits, eligibility, or Medicare beneficiary cost sharing (including Parts A and B premiums); or result in a change in the beneficiary premium percentage or low-income subsidies under Part D. Hospitals and hospices (through 2019) and clinical labs (for one year) will not be subject to cost reductions proposed by the board. The board must also submit recommendations every other year to slow the growth in national health expenditures while preserving quality of care by January 1, 2015. One does not envy the task of the Payment Advisory Board.

A summary of major proposals made by national commissions and prominent public figures in the past two years can be found in the Bipartisan Policy Center report: "Side-by-Side Comparison to Simpson Bowles Commission," (BPC Domenici-Rivlin Task Force, President Obama, and Chairman Ryan). Most of the proposals lay the problem at the feet of the fee-for-service approach in Medicare. Fundamental to this view is the conviction that a public program this large and complex is beyond the management capabilities of mere humans. Hence, the bringing to the fore of market-based solutions. Variations on this theme have included:

Roadmap for America's Future Act of 2010 (Rep. Paul Ryan legislation, 27 January 2010)

Restoring America's Future (The Debt Reduction Task Force, Senator Pete Domenici and Dr. Alice Rivlin, co-chairs, Bipartisan Policy Center, November 2010)

A Longterm Plan for Medicare and Medicaid ("Rivlin-Ryan" proposal to the Simpson/Bowles Commission, November 2010)

Path to Prosperity (Rep. Paul Ryan Budget Proposal for FY2012)

These argue for partial or complete transition of Medicare from a fee-for-service to a premium support (or voucher) system. The primary articulated differences among them are the beginning date, the method to determine the initial support level, and the rate at which that support level increases. All mention adjustments in levels of support (e.g., for income level, health status, age) for individuals within a cohort, with the exception of the *Ryan Path to Prosperity*, and yet they are all vague as to specifics.

The Domenici-Rivlin plan is the "most generous" in allowed annual increase in per capita support (GDP +1%) and in permitting traditional Medicare fee-for-service to continue as an option, but subject to increased premiums if the overall GDP + 1% goal is not maintained. The *Ryan Path to Prosperity* is the least generous in the allowed rate-of-increase of the basic premium support (consumer price index-urban) and in discontinuing fee-for-service Medicare for those whose age was 55 and under in 2010.

As all of the proposals are aimed at reducing the growth rate of federal spending for Medicare, all can be expected to depress benefits in the aggregate unless remarkable market efficiencies emerge. The one plan having sufficient specificity for the Congressional Budget Office to assess future impact on individuals is the *Ryan Budget Proposal*. Specifically, the CBO asked first, what would a standard health care package cost if covered either under traditional Medicare or under the Ryan plan and, second, what portion of those (different) costs would be borne by the individual?

In its analysis, the CBO used its alternative fiscal scenario, a projection based on the realistic assumption that annual Congressional "patches" (e.g., for the alternative minimum tax, physician reimbursement under Medicare, et al.) will continue to be the (irresponsible?) pattern. Its conclusions:

> In 2022, *if* the cost of the standard package under the Ryan plan were "$100," the cost under Medicare would be $72. Under Ryan, the individual would bear a cost of $62 to purchase the $100 plan. Under Medicare the individual would bear a cost of $30 for the equivalent $72 plan.
>
> In 2030, the comparative numbers for the "$100" standard would be a Medicare cost of $71, with the amounts borne by the individual being $68 under Ryan and $30 under Medicare.

The CBO is clear in stating that these numbers are anything but hard. Quite plausibly, however, the CBO concludes:

> Under the proposal, the gradually increasing number of Medicare beneficiaries participating in the new premium support program would bear a much larger share of their health care costs than they would under the traditional program. That greater burden would require them to reduce their use of health care services, spend less on other goods and services, or save more in advance of retirement than they would under current law.

Note: In December, 2011, a new proposal was offered by Senator Ron Wyden (D-Oregon) and Paul Ryan (R-Wisconsin). Its main feature would allow traditional Medicare fee-for-service to continue alongside a premium-support plan. Seemingly, this modification is designed to soften some of the harsher criticism that has been directed at the *Ryan Path to Prosperity*. We do not review that proposal here.

Our "Healthy Normal Aging" Proposal

We agree that fee-for-service Medicare must be reformed. However, we assert that the role of elders in reform must be better articulated and the costs they are asked to bear made clearer as a matter of policy, not emerging as the accidental outcome of the market. Laying down an arbitrary goal, as in the Patient Protection and Affordable Care Act, and asking an advisory board to derive an impossible solution is not an answer. Further, to propose market solutions without delineating their impact on individuals falls short. One can commend Representative Ryan for being sufficiently specific that the partial CBO analysis of impact was possible.

We assert that an informed discussion involving those who will be affected is needed. This discussion must also include the role of those of us who typically are offered the plum of escaping any negative effects of the changes. We are all in this together. First, that means we must become well versed on the subject. The internet is rife with information on the topic, unfortunately most often from a highly biased viewpoint. There are good sources of information but a critical eye is required. Second, we recommend Fast Facts, a web compilation of slides prepared by The Henry J. Kaiser Family Foundation, and The Dartmouth Atlas of Health Care, a statistical display of information gathered from the 306 Hospital Referral Regions in the U.S. These two sources provide great detail and considerable insight in an easy-to-grasp format. Listed below are sample facts highly relevant to the question of cost and affordability.

From The Dartmouth Atlas of Health Care (Dartmouth):

> There is very significant variation in the expenditure levels among the Hospital Referral Regions (HHRs). In 2007, the expenditure per beneficiary for the HHR at the median of the most cost-efficient quintile was $7,087 per year compared to $9,765 for the median HHR of the least cost-efficient quintile.
>
> Chronic-disease care is a huge part of Medicare expenditures, during the period 2003–2007 amounting to 75% of the total. End-of-life (final two years) chronic care by itself was 32% of the total.

According to Fast Facts (KFF):

KFF provides a slightly different angle. In 2006, 58% of total Medicare expenditures were devoted to 10% of the beneficiaries. The average annual cost for that group was $48,210 per beneficiary compared to $3,910 for the remaining 90%.

Drawing on the CBO Baseline Projection, the estimate for expenditures on pharmaceuticals is projected to rise from 11% of total spending to 19% of a much larger total in 2020.

In 2006, the average out-of-pocket costs to the beneficiary (premiums, deductibles, and co-pays) were $4,241; for those over age 85 the amount was $7,487. On average, out-of-pocket costs were 16% of income.

Income statistics in 2006: Median income per beneficiary was $22,800; 21% had incomes greater than $40,000 and 33% had incomes below 150% of the federal poverty level.

To advance the discussion of what should be considered, we lay out a general program we feel is in consonance with our earlier prescription for Healthy Normal Aging. It is configured to allow freedom of choice to the individual: a privatized premium-support option, a combination public and private option, and for the true libertarians, no option at all. The program is summarized below.

Summary of the Healthy Normal Aging Proposal

The Private Option

The private option is a premium-support plan to provide individual choice for any approved health-care plan subject to its availability and affordability. The objective of this option would be to maximize consumers' freedom. It follows the philosophy of Representative Ryan's proposals.

It would establish a nationwide insurance exchange from which individuals at age 65 could use their premium subsidy to purchase a private policy.

Only policies approved for the exchange would qualify for the subsidy. To be listed, a policy could not exclude coverage of pre-existing conditions or allow cancellation for new circumstances for individuals entering the program. A policy's terms must be uniform for all covered.

The initial upper limit on the premium support would be set based on historical costs for Medicare as of that time. The upper limit would change annually according to a prescribed cost index.

For each calendar year, those reaching age 65 would be assigned to a new cohort. For each cohort, the initial limit on the premium support would be reset in the light of the most recent general health care cost trends. Thereafter, the limit would change by the prescribed cost index. There would be a trial period extending for two years after first eligibility during which the individual would be free to defer date of initial enrollment and/or to transfer to the public/private option with no restrictions. After the trial period, individuals could enroll in the private option or transfer to the public/private option but with the prospect of losing coverage for pre-existing conditions not covered by a previous plan.

The Public/Private Option

The objective of the public/private option would be to provide care in consonance with the concept of Healthy Normal Aging. That includes acknowledging that as age-related health care costs increase, the individual ought to assume a greater share of the economic burden. It comprises three interlocking components:

1. **Acute care**, a fee-for-service plan with a limited maximum coverage per year. The plan would be oriented to acute-, preventive-, restorative- and ameliorative-care. It would have no annual enrollment fee and no deductibles, but would include income-related co-payments.
2. **Limited major medical**, individual policies purchased from the nationwide insurance exchange. Policies offered on the exchange would receive premium support related to the income of the individual. To be listed on the exchange, a policy would be required to begin coverage of expenses at the upper limit of the Acute Care component and to meet specified minimum standards. A government-provided plan meeting the specified minimum standards would be offered at an appropriate price. Private policies on the exchange would be allowed to exceed the specified minimum standards.
3. **Public major medical**, a final shield for the individual against extremely high-cost non-elective procedures. It would have no annual enrollment fee and no co-payments.

An individual choosing to enroll in the public/private option initially would be required to sign on to all three components. After a specified number of years, continuation in Limited Major Medical would become optional.

As with the private option, the first two years of the Public Option would be a trial period; following that period the individual would be free to change policies and options, subject to the proviso on pre-existing conditions.

The public/private option is described in greater detail in Appendix B. with a specific hypothetical example to illustrate the nature of its impact on individuals.

Uninsured Individuals and Extreme Hardship Cases

A vexing problem for any voluntary market-based support program is the individual who, for good reasons or bad, chooses not to maintain insurance that is subsequently needed. It is, simply, a fact of life that members of our society do not care to spend money for something they do not like or for which they (hope to) have no need. (This writer pleads guilty on that account for insurance to cover longterm assisted care.)

What is to be done when an unaffordable problem strikes an uninsured individual?

First rule: Appropriate emergency care is always provided and paid for with public funds if no other alternative is available.

Second rule: In non-emergency situations, appropriate medical procedures will not be denied a patient who requests them, with the proviso that the patient understands the financial consequences.

Third rule: A plan will be set up whereby the individual will pay in time what he or she is able from income and assets.

The procedure for covering expenses might be similar in concept to disaster aid. The patient, after appropriately drawing down liquid assets, would be granted a loan to be repaid by any of a number of mechanisms; e.g., reverse mortgages for owner-occupied housing, liens against other non-liquid assets, affordable payments, claims against estates, etc. The spirit of the arrangement would follow the lead of the existing procedure for Medicaid support of longterm assisted living. The message: "You will not be denied treatment, but the economic consequences to you and/or your heirs may not be what you would like."

The above "disaster aid" concept, suitably modified, would apply to cases deemed as extreme hardship.

Financial Clarity in the Process

We believe that self-restraints on expenditures produced by out-of-pocket costs are greatly reduced in effectiveness because of obscurity. For one, these costs and the charges on which the costs are assigned are typically not identified until long after the fact. Further, Medicare suffers from a disease similar to that of the supermarket industry in touting "How much you have saved" (but from a highly suspect price base), only in a much more obscure format.

We believe information technology in the digital age is capable of giving immediate information to the doctor and patient on the probable or final cost of the large bulk of treatment components that may be considered. This implies that, for services provided in the public/private option, standards ought to be established and kept current for most routine procedures, tests, and pharmaceuticals. There is no good reason why, back in 2006, I should not have been informed at the time a doctor scheduled an MRI on my shoulder that it would cost $800, with a $160 co-pay. I care about both. When more complex questions arise, there must be an immediate opportunity for consultation with a knowledgeable professional. We suggest establishing such professional disciplines as part of hospital services.

Tort reform: We recommend that tort reform of a reasonable sort should be established for practitioners in the public/private option. We leave to others what that might be.

Sharing the burden: A "divide and conquer" mentality should not be accepted. If there must be give in order to achieve a more reasonable health care program, we must all participate. We assert that any reform program must include assigning an appropriate share of the cost burden to those who otherwise might escape because of age.

Public funding: We do not address the mechanism for public funding for the overall program. We remain largely silent on the issue of how current private assessments (i.e., FICA taxes, Parts B and D premiums, deductibles, and co-payments) are to be melded into the program. We do suggest that it is time to consider a large-scale national reformation of transfer payments (an unfortunately politically pejorative term) involving the individual. Given the information management capabilities that have emerged in the digital age, it would seem to make eminent sense to integrate Social Security and Medicare with the Internal Revenue Service. This also would be the occasion to abandon the fiction that levying FICA taxes is for the purposes of saving for individual pensions or purchasing an individual health insurance policy. The origin of this notion derived from what Franklin Delano Roosevelt saw as necessary political protection of a, then-revolutionary, concept. One would hope that we as a nation have moved beyond that need, though recent political discourse does raise some doubt.

Personal Things to Remember

12

The Importance of Humor, Domestic Pets, Music and Interpersonal Relationships

Humor is an important part of aging. The main point is to keep a sense of it or, if you lost it along the way, to get it back. For example, in the author's environment one is not allowed to celebrate a birthday if the potential celebrant is over 40 years of age. The author realized that each time he had a birthday he became a year older. Therefore, there will be no more birthday parties. The reasoning was based on the idea that an old calendar, invented by Cesar Augustus thousands of years ago, should not be the determining factor as to when a person is getting older. He tried to change to the Chinese calendar, but that offered no help either. Then, he remembered the Gilbert and Sullivan operetta, *Pirates of Penzance*, in which the young man could not get his reward at age 21 because he was born on February 29th. There must be another way to emerge into the elder group than by a calendar.

Domestic Animal Companions

A great deal of consideration and research has been given to the notion of whether or not to have a domestic pet—a cat or a dog. Research has shown that elders, particularly those living alone, have healthier and longer lives if they share their existence with a dog or a cat. We are sure this is true. One reason is that, as we grow older, our circle of existence gets smaller. Friends slip away and we become more insular and introverted. At this time, a furry friend, like a cat on the lap, becomes a wonderful addition to our lives. A dog can provide a great reason for us to go out for a walk several times a day—adding to our health and also enhancing the likelihood of our meeting people along the way. Pets may also provide a valuable service in warning us of danger from unusual odors, like leaking gas, or intruders, and they can help guide us along our walks or possibly fetch slippers or a newspaper.

Music

Another thing that keeps us young is music. No matter how old one gets, music can be invigorating and enjoyable, as well as capable of widening our experience. Even better than listening is playing an instrument or singing—it requires effort, practice, and focused attention, all of which can improve our brain function. This has been made especially easy because technology allows us to play or sing along with the greatest choruses or orchestras in the world simply by placing a CD in the player (or loading a song on our computer or handheld music-playing device, for those of us really up to date with technology) and turning up the volume. You do not have to be a great musician so long as you enjoy yourself. The author knew a fellow who loved to sing—particularly Beethoven's Ninth Symphony—but he had trouble carrying a tune. So when the spirit moved him, he would go out to his car, put on the CD player and sing his heart out! Electric pianos with headphones allow the same opportunity without any concern about intruding on others or hitting a clunker once in awhile. There are countless ways we can each enjoy music. Consider attending concerts or borrowing CDs from the library.

The author began playing the cello at 55 years of age. After 10 years of lessons and practice, he was good enough to join an amateur orchestra (see below—the bearded man in the cello section—the oldest member of the Basel, Switzerland, TriRhenum Orchestra). This author learned, even late in life, how much fun it is to be surrounded by music, practice, music lessons, and friends during rehearsals.

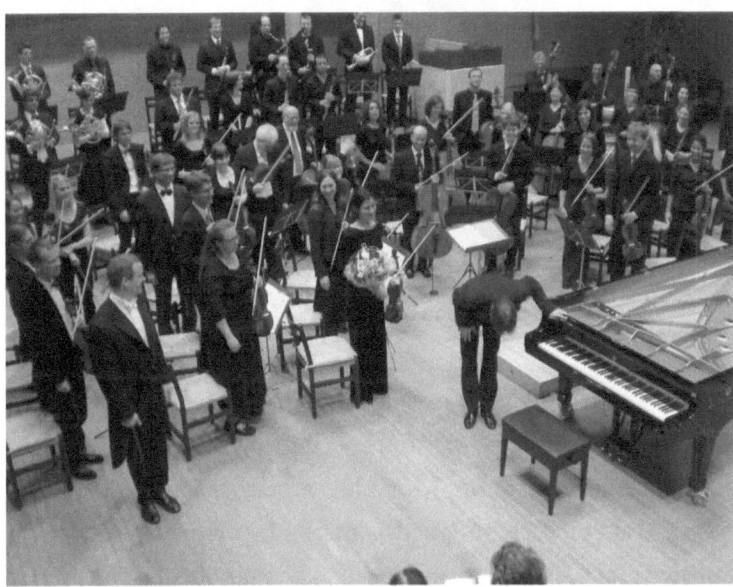

Figure 5. The author in the cello section of the TriRhenum Orchestra.

There are professional psychologists who provide music therapy for their patients. One can easily order CDs that can be used for meditation, exercise programs, and just for background enjoyment. Jacqueline Stohler, a flutist and music therapist at St. Clara hospital in Switzerland, uses a Klangbett in music therapy. The Klangbett is a soundbed specially constructed with 56 harp strings attached to the under surface of the bed. By playing these strings as one would play a harp, the therapist provides comfort to the patient.

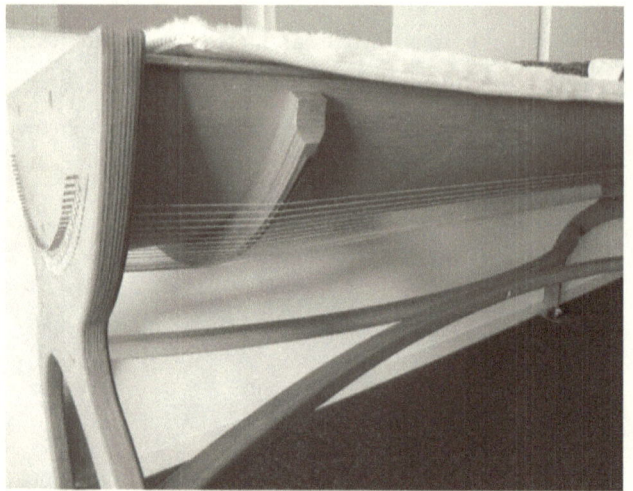

Figure 6. The Klangbett (soundbed).

Music therapy is a psycho-therapeutic method in which, by either actively playing music (improvisation) or passively receiving music (listening), psychic processes can be supported and accompanied. Through this method, personal resources are activated and creativity is enhanced. The soundbed is one of many musical instruments that are used in music therapy. Patients can perceive both the sound and the vibration, and most feel relaxation through a feeling of emotional security and a reduction of anxiety and easing of pain.

Another example of music therapy is the use of an instrument called a Miltone 1. This instrument has eight tones that can be played by hand or with a mallet by either the therapist or the patient. For periods of about 10 to 15 minutes, the Miltone provides a soothing source of sound. The gong is also a useful instrument, but it has a different purpose. It provides those with aggressive tendencies or anger, a temporary outlet to relieve tension or frustration.

Hand-in-hand with music is dance. Many elders enjoy the social outlet and exercise that accompany dancing—whether it be group movement as part of an organized class, square dancing, line dancing, or ballroom dancing enjoyed with partners. Dancing is exercise; exercise generates pheromones in the brain that are known to create a sense of enjoyment and well-being.

These examples should remind us that music and dance are wonderful ways to experience life in general, and wonderful ways to emerge into the elder population with a rich tradition to call upon at any time.

Interpersonal Relationships

Another important part of living a fulfilling life is our various interpersonal relationships. As in most 21st-century books, we cannot—nor should we—avoid the subject of elder sexual identity. How we handle the issue of relationships and sex as we age is a challenge—not because we are unable or uninterested, but because we are of a generation that did not openly discuss the subject and so we are now left with questions many of us are hesitant to ask. Our thoughts and fantasies about sex do not vanish with age—in fact, they may grow stronger while our bodies may be challenged to keep up.

As physicians who have been practicing medicine for many years, we were seldom required to deal with this issue—our patients were hesitant to broach the subject and we likely had little to offer if they did. The wretched stereotypes attached to sex and elders are thankfully waning—we all remember too well the infamous photo of the old man with his raincoat open with the banner, "Expose yourself to art!" or the often-used derogatory phrase about ". . . dirty old men" or the image of the fading movie star clinging to youth in the film *Sunset Boulevard*. Happily, those images are changing and are being replaced by phrases like, "Sixty is the new 50 . . . seventy is the new 60 . . ." and we can enjoy images of a radiant, fit Jane Fonda in her 70s. There are more television physicians, like Dr. Oz, who encourage all of us to get more exercise and stay active, which helps us all to thrive, not merely survive, including having a healthy sex life.

As physicians, we strongly recommend that elders avoid the dangers of seeking out prostitutes. Such activities pose health problems from venereal diseases and other sexually transmitted diseases, and they are demeaning to the prostitutes, to the individuals making the payments, and to their extended families.

Recently, in a city in Switzerland, an 87-year-old woman became tired of noisy prostitutes plying their trade on the sidewalk beneath her apartment windows. To combat the intrusion on her peace and quiet, or perhaps to send a message to the paying customers that they would be better off seeking more appropriate company elsewhere, she poured water from a small green watering can over the side of her terrace onto the ladies of the night. Apparently, she had quite good aim and repeated the practice frequently. The police were called and told her to stop but she apparently proved that she was breaking no existing law. She is now infamous as "the lady who makes the prostitutes wet." This may be another example of aging aggressively.

Putting aside the possibility of domestic violence, inappropriate public displays, frequenting prostitutes, or chasing after men or women who might be inappropriate for our stage in life, what should our message about sexual activity be?

We strongly advocate reinforcing our fantasies with a liberal dose of reminiscing—especially if we are lucky enough to be with a longtime partner. Holding hands or caressing with your favorite person, taking the time to go on a "date" with the person you may tend to take for granted, planning a romantic outing or trip, or going to a movie and sharing a bag of popcorn . . . all of these are ways to enhance our intimate relationship with the person we care about. Give these ideas a try if you have forgotten or, worse, if you think the time for such things has passed with age. We are still alive—that means we are not too old for romance.

My wife and I recently watched a film entitled, *New York, I Love You.* The film contains a number of vignettes written by New Yorkers about the city they love. One of the scenes featured a long-married couple walking along a boardwalk next to the sea. It was poignant and touching to see them enjoying each other as they thought about their long lives together in the city they loved. Young people may plan their future joys, but one of the beauties of aging is that we can share our good memories with each other.

As physicians, we can recommend several things. If you are involved in a sexual relationship with a significant other, do not stop; if you want to be and you are not, due to fear or feelings of physical inadequacy, men should discuss this with their primary physician and women should speak with their gynecologists. The matter of sexuality and aging is no longer taboo and these physicians are well equipped to provide guidance and support. In the meantime, you might consider a few commonsense guidelines.

First and foremost, for both good health and romance, good daily hygiene is a must. Some elders have a tendency to let daily showering, shaving, hair trimming, dressing, and so on, fall by the wayside. Do not let this happen. Personal hygiene is as important to our health as exercise, and possibly more important for the purpose of an intimate relationship.

Second, in case you have forgotten, watch a good movie to remind yourself about how to woo the person you want to be with—yes, woo. We are never too old for a little romance in our day-to-day lives. There is a lovely scene in the movie *Moonstruck*, when an older couple is carried away by the light of the moon and a reminiscence from their youth—the next day while they are working in their little grocery store, it is obvious they spent a romantic night together that they can revel in.

We are never too old to pay our partner a compliment or bring home flowers or plan an evening out. And even simpler, but equally important, is sharing a newspaper article you know will interest your significant other, or making a new photo album together . . . the list is endless. It has been statistically proven that a warm and loving relationship is the best prescription for a healthier, longer life. If you have lost a loved one, get out of your house and rejoin the world.

If you follow our basic advice, you may find that life holds some new and unexpected opportunities. If you have a life partner, rekindle a little romance and keep the flame burning.

13

Memories are an important part of aging—Both the Good and the Bad

As we age, both good and bad memories become a part of our everyday activities—our decision making, our dreams, our frustration or joy at events occurring in our daily lives are all affected by our experiences that are now memories.

The Bad Ones First—The War in Vietnam 1967–1969

This author cannot watch a movie or television program that portrays reality or fantasy about the Vietnam War of the 1960s or early 1970s. After being drafted, he chose to drive to basic training in Texas. He planned to put his automobile on a freighter so he could have it while he worked in an army hospital in the Philippines. Two years of his life committed to the United States Air Force seemed like a long time, but he approached it with resignation that most young people caught up in the Vietnam conflict had accepted. He was glad that he was a physician; somehow it meant he did not have to face the moral decision others had to face: to kill for an ill-defined, opportunistic national cause or to reject the nation's commitment and refuse to serve in the military, as some of his friends had done.

As a physician, he could rationalize that he would be caring for the health of the young men who had accepted the assignment. If they were reluctant to continue their part in the nightmare, he would find a way to make their disease or injury more significant for the records; if they really wanted to continue in battle with their comrades, then he would help them get well as rapidly as possible.

In any case, during his long solo drive to Texas, he was impressed that the country he had just been hired to defend was a big one. This observation helped him blunt his outward and continuous internal opposition to the United States involvement in the War—the United States was worth a great deal and he could do his part.

The author's life was changing in a dramatic fashion. He was leaving the protective walls of medical training programs and heading for an unknown world. He stopped smoking, began to exercise, and he developed a pattern of mental organization in order to deal with the challenges ahead. At the basic training camp in Texas, he learned a lot about being a soldier. Even on the pistol range he realized that, in spite of being a doctor, he was being prepared for war. Later, as bleeding, terribly wounded, and often ill young men came under his care, he would recall those feelings at the shooting range. Impersonal was the theme—these youths had been damaged, sometimes destroyed by an awful, non-human force called war.

He spent two years feeling the complete conflict between a human healer and an inhuman force. During those two years, he aged—he lost his boyhood optimism and began to see life day by day as the present plus a little past, but not a future. Like thousands of others, after those two years and for the rest of his life he could not accept any statement that included the phrase, "The war was honorable, necessary or useful . . ." from anyone. War is a form of hell that no human deserves.

After those two years, the author realized that Vietnam had done many important and painful things to him. He had matured but, even though he returned to the United States with a wife and three children, he really felt he had returned home alone. Like many others who returned from the Vietnam experience, he was unable to share his experiences with anyone.

Back in the United States, he began his life of research and teaching but his family life fell apart. For many years, he lived his life as a teacher, traveler, and researcher—it was fulfilling, but incomplete. This would change years later, but the Vietnam War and its effect on his life remain with him until today.

In subsequent years, there were other bad memories from which he will never recover—watching children dying of measles in a Cambodian refugee camp on the Thailand border (Thai authorities would not allow use of measles vaccine in the refugee camp because it was not available to their own local Thai farmers in the same region). The meningitis epidemic in the camp of 100,000 displaced persons caused suffering from the same thinking process, even though farmers spread over hundreds of miles would not have had the same disease patterns as in a crowded refugee camp. These bad memories come from a sense of helplessness—maybe not too dissimilar from the author's present feelings about the Medicare and Medicaid health crisis in the United States.

The Good times—1983 to the Present

Perhaps, to help him recover from the bad times, this author found his long ago college sweetheart. He found her in Switzerland, where she had been living with her family. Despite their years apart, the creation of their own families, and some difficult years for them both, their romance remained strong. They continued to make new plans for their life together.

The task was daunting. First, he managed to arrange a sabbatical year at the Microbiology Institute in Basle, requiring him to fly back and forth every few months to meet his teaching and consulting obligations at Cornell University Medical College in New York. After a year, the author and his girlfriend knew that they had to take the next step. The author went through the arduous task of applying for a position as Medical Expert in the Clinical Section at Sandoz Pharmaceutical Company in Basle—and his application was accepted. He had to resign his post as professor of medicine and chief of international medicine, leaving his academic career and friends and colleagues behind. He and Madeleine were married with only his mother present at an intimate wedding ceremony in his hometown of Medina, Ohio. The new couple went to the Caribbean for a weeklong honeymoon—a mistake they soon realized since neither of them enjoyed sitting on the beach or sailing or eating hotel food. Back in Basle on January 1, 1986, the author started his new career.

The next 25 years of life with a new life partner, in a different culture, speaking a new language and learning the new roles of husband and clinical researcher are difficult to summarize. For the most part, life was tranquil and a delight. The author's new work was demanding—there was so much to learn about designing clinical trials (the author had been a physician and teacher and had done basic research in a laboratory setting). He had to learn data collection, how to discuss trial results with pharmaceutical executives with drug development in mind; then make certain that those in the Swiss national regulatory agencies and those in the Sandoz-affiliated companies all over the world had enough information to adequately communicate that new information to physicians using the drugs Sandoz produced.

The author had traveled extensively in his previous life to national and international medical conferences, and to more distant locales in the world where he taught young doctors and provided medical care in refugee camps. Now traveling was different. Tom's wife accompanied him—they spent several weeks in many parts of China, they traveled to Taiwan, Singapore, Hong Kong, Nepal, Brazil, Russia, Finland, and nearly every major city in Europe, where he lectured on infectious diseases and on the new drugs designed to treat skin infections. The author also traveled to some more remote places, like Kazakhstan, alone. He served as a medical advisor to the World Health Organization and went to Central Africa to discuss meningococcal meningitis, and to Tajikistan to make recommendations about the typhoid fever epidemic there.

In retrospect, we can see that we were passing through the phases of our lives and our marriage that we would subsequently describe to our children: the first phase of lustful love; the second phase of succeeding in our professional lives while running a home, planning for our financial futures, helping our children; and now the more companionable phase of mostly leaving work behind and enjoying more of our life together. The current phase, though perhaps not as exciting as the first two phases, is fully enjoyable for us both.

This author has spent some time thinking about the day that one of them will no longer be living. He wants to be the first to go because he knows his wife will be much better able to handle a solo life than he would. Of course, they have done what we hope all the readers of this book have done—made the necessary preparations for financial security for both of them. They have also discussed issues such as proper nursing care as needed, moving to an apartment with an elevator, how to enjoy stress-free vacations, and how to best ensure the soft landing discussed in chapter 2.

He is also part of the Celtic tradition that believes when he leaves life as we know it, he will be on a ship sailing to the Isle of Avalon to be with his ancestors. His mother and father will be there and he will be held tightly by his father, with his father's three sisters, Carol, Ann, and Mary, standing close by. There will also be little Maggie, his daughter Phoebe's daughter who passed on when only a baby— she will be playing happily with all of the other children, each taken too soon from this earth. There is no disease or illness on Avalon. Of course, this is the author's vision—each one reading this book will have a vision of his or her own that can provide comfort as we move along our life's course.

This chapter has been presented in a very personal way so that the reader will be empowered to examine his or her own memories. Those memories are a part of each of our lives and, as we age, they occupy a more dominant role in our consciousness. Do not allow yourself the pain of pretending they do not exist. Though sometimes painful to recall, our memories are wonderful and should be shared with our families and those we care most about.

Conclusion

14

Aging is A Wonderful Process But It Must Be Done Aggressively

The great thing about getting older is that we gain a new and freeing perspective—things that once seemed so important are not so important after all. For example, surviving the teen years, the first kiss, getting through school, finding a job, feeling fulfilled—it is so nice not to worry about all that stuff.

Your author has been among the lucky ones—he had the opportunity to establish good relationships with his children and can spend sufficient attention on his grandchildren; he was able to get his finances in order and ensure he had a pension; and he has been able to make the right choices to foster his overall health. He feels that the aggression of life and for life has been fun and should not stop because of a few aches and pains, or because a younger generation thinks they can do what he has done better—they cannot mainly because they need more experience to even begin to compete!

We hope you have received the message that the concept of aging as a gradual, but inevitable, process of decline is totally inaccurate. It is now clear that such perceived decline has been due to health care planners and politicians looking for information in all the wrong places. They have been looking at nursing homes and retirement centers where isolation and absent mental and physical stimulation give the perception of decline, rather than looking at the places where elders are active and creative. When the correct data are collected, there is little evidence for any age-related decline.

Writing this book has enabled us to examine the various approaches of local, state, and federal governments in the United States and to try to determine how this structure has affected the well-being of society. As you have read through this book, perhaps you have come to the same realization as your author, contributor, and editor: the current state of health care in the United States is a failure, bordering now on a total crisis. The problem is very clear— the majority of the United States population does not want to pay the amount of money needed to provide universal health care, and the period of borrowing the needed funds is over. The United States is a democracy and this is the choice of the majority—it has been the choice for decades—so it should not be a surprise that we have reached this impasse now that our collective heads have hit the debt ceiling again.

Medicare and Medicaid resources are diminishing rapidly, personal health insurance plans are inadequate and filled with corruption; the choice for the future appears to depend entirely on each individual's mixture of personal finances, credit lines, and family support. Only as individuals can we make the necessary decisions to ensure the financial security needed to protect us from illness, immobility, and isolation as we grow older. We urge you all to examine your individual status now and make the difficult decisions immediately, and we wish us all good luck.

Afterword

Some of the fun of putting this book together has been observing how aging people—the author, the contributing author (John Cotton), John and Lynda Burton, and the editor (Betsy Chalfin)—became so feisty while debating each concept and paragraph. There certainly has been no sign of age-related decline—except perhaps in the perceived stubbornness of us elders! Another part of the fun has been interacting with our brothers, sisters, wives, husbands, children, grandchildren, and friends while having them help us obtain the vital information needed and conveying it with the greatest possible accuracy. Maybe each family should work on a family book filled with creative ideas just to see how much fun each generation can bring to the discussion. We hope this book provides a few others with the foresight (or luck) we have had in planning for our long and active and aggressive futures.

Appendices

Appendix A

Confusing Language is a Major Problem in Understanding Medication for Young and Old

The preceding chapters may have given the impression that we are against the use of medication for elders. This is not the case. However, we do insist that prescribed medications be properly tested in the cohort of people to whom a particular medication is administered, not in some other group. Making sure beneficial medications become available to the public is a problem because of the difficulty in designing a proper clinical drug trial in the first place. Here we demonstrate how statistics can be manipulated so that they determine the trial design and its results instead of answering the important question of how the drug will work for an individual patient.

Clinical Trial Design and Statistical Analysis

The process used to determine whether a certain drug is safe and effective for use by humans has comprised a long history of pharmaceutical development and government regulatory procedures. The steps in studying a new drug are complex, expensive, and time consuming. Two statistical procedures have been vital in this process: 1) rejecting the null hypothesis in order to prove superiority of a new drug or procedure over the existing treatment; and 2) documenting statistical equivalence of two drugs or procedures by use of confidence limits. These two procedures determine whether a drug is to be recommended by physicians, medical societies, pharmaceutical companies, and governments. The point made here is that neither procedure addresses a patient's quality of life when he or she is advised to take a drug shown statistically to be effective.

Rejecting the null hypothesis as a device in drug trials was adopted over 60 years ago as a compromise in data analysis. There are many other ways to conclude that one intervention is better than another, but statisticians decided that the simplest method was best and therefore adopted the rejection of the null hypothesis. This means that one assumes that two interventions are similar (i.e., null) and that one must reject their similarity by showing they are different. But how different is different?

It was decided that if the difference could be due to random events, then they were not different. This was the first problem. An arbitrary decision was made to say that, if there was a shift of 5% between the two groups being tested (defined as a p value of 0.05 or less) then the one intervention was more valuable than the other (i.e., not a random event). Another arbitrary decision stated that, to use this method, only one outcome could be examined (the primary efficacy parameter). If the study met the criteria of rejecting the null hypothesis looking at the primary efficacy parameter, the intervention could be considered useful. The process became more complicated by insisting that this rejection process not only apply to a carefully balanced group study of the intervention and dose limitations (i.e., Phase II studies), but would also be seen in larger studies of all sorts of people that might meet the entry criteria for use of the intervention (i.e., Phase III studies). Based on this data, the intervention tested was approved by regulatory agencies and then the drug or procedure could be used in humans.

At the end of all this, we consumers had an arbitrary statistical endpoint and a large study group but it was not possible to evaluate whether the intervention was important to the quality of our lives. Why not? Because no measurement of that quality was available. That decision was left to the primary physician because only he or she could translate all of the information and apply the facts to the individual patient. But what tools were provided to help make that decision?

Our answer to that question, and the reason for this appendix, is that physicians are given hardly any tools—information nor legal representation to defend them, if they decide not to prescribe a specific drug, nor independent advertising to present their point of view. The common perception among physicians has become, "... if I, as the primary care provider, do not provide this heavily advertised drug, my patient will simply go to someone else who will provide it . . ." We must aggressively demand the resources to educate both physicians and patients.

Misusing language in clinical trial design and statistical analysis is characterized not so much by labeling errors of the process but by misunderstanding what is truly being sought when a clinical trial is planned. Clinical trials can have many different objectives, so their planning should state and reflect the specific objective of a given trial. At the present time, that is not the case.

A clinical trial done in a university-based medical center, when no sponsor is likely to gain by the results of the trial, may ask a question like, "Does a certain approach to patient care actually benefit the patient?" Depending on the complexity of the approach being examined, the trial may have to be single-blinded, double-blinded, or it could be open-label or observational. The key part of the above sentence, the part that has made the conduct of clinical trials so confusing as a result of mislabeling, is the statement, ". . . with no sponsor likely to gain by the results of the trial." Actually, there are very few clinical trials done in which no one gains by the results, but the types of gain are so varied or ignored that the clinical trials process suffers and, ultimately, health care suffers as well.

While employed at a university (and funded by federal grants or patient care), we could design and publish all sorts of observations about patient care without much attention to questions like: were observations being made on a random population (almost never); were some patients excluded from the analysis because of complicating issues not associated with the question being studied (almost always); was someone, including those conducting the study, likely to benefit by the results of the study (almost certainly).

The benefits attained by those conducting the research included: presenting interesting conclusions at national and international meetings, thus improving their status among their peers; publishing study results, thus improving one's curriculum vitae, affecting promotions in the university; increasing the likelihood of success when competing for grants (successful research outcomes under a currently funded grant looks good on grant applications); not to mention the possibility that the study might attract needed pharmaceutical interest for a department's fellowship funding in the future. The only potential bias we had to record in publications was whether we owned stock in any related company at the time the study was published. If the information presented was borderline or inconclusive, we gained little; if it was dramatic, we (and the university) gained a great deal. Did all of the potential benefits to the study designers or to our universities allow bias to enter the study? Almost certainly! We likely would not have bothered spending our time doing the study if we were not quite certain that the results would be as predicted. That alone appears to be an impressive bias.

When the author was fully employed by a pharmaceutical company, the change in clinical trial design was dramatic. Now, everything done was examined with the highest level of scrutiny and suspicion since the researcher, or actually the company, might gain financially. The approach to trial design was different for several reasons: 1) there was no reward in bonus or higher salary because of a successful clinical trial; 2) these trials seldom complimented ones curriculum vitae—in fact, the pharmaceutical company researcher was often not even included as an author on a resulting publication, even though he or she designed the trial; 3) the researcher's salary was secure and less dependent on the clinical trial than it was for those at a university; and 4) pharmaceutical companies gained very little (and sometimes lost a lot) by presenting data erroneously—the most common reason to massage data was to overcome errors in trial design, not to try to prove that an ineffective drug was effective.

The main difference between clinical research at a university and a pharmaceutical company is that in the latter clinical trials are a routine component of the bureaucratic and heavily supervised regulatory process. It is the entry into this process that dramatically changes the design and meaning of a clinical trial. Phases of clinical trial conduct were still referred to by the numbers I through IV, but now they had a regulatory meaning, not a medical research meaning. It is also clear that the words "clinical trial" have a variety of meanings or scientific interpretation in the practice of medicine.

In a recent book chapter summarizing some newer thoughts about the use of clinical trials, the author pointed out that although only randomized-controlled clinical trials (so-called "evidence-based" clinical trials) were of importance in the drug registration process, only 20% of physicians considered these results when making their prescribing decisions.

The discussion in that article was meant as a criticism of the information process that does not convey the true message to practicing physicians. Of course, that is not the problem. The problem is that clinical trials have no meaning for the physician because they are observations on groups of patients that produce statistical information that is of almost no value to a physician with a single patient who has a very individual problem. Randomized trials are often less relevant to a physician's thinking and judgment than are open-label drug trial experiences, opinions of leaders in the field, or anecdotal personal experience.

It is clear that what one group considers to be the ideal standard for a clinical trial is often considered of borderline value by another group. A major problem is the misunderstanding between the scientists, statisticians, and regulatory affairs people on one hand, and health care providers on the other. The former tend to think the latter are unintelligent or uninformed, or both. They think that what a physician needs is simple instructions on how to use drugs, primarily based on information from properly done clinical trials. In reality, health care providers are over-informed and, out of politeness or a lack of time, they select their own sources to guide their judgments concerning patient care—and in a recent study only 20% thought the advice based on randomized-controlled clinical trials was appropriate for their decision-making process! This comes as such a shock to policymakers that, of course, the physicians are labeled as incompetent!

Appendix B

A Conceptual Societal Health Program for Elders

The following is an approach for a health-care program consistent with the principles of Healthy Normal Aging described in chapter 2 and previewed in chapter 11. It is conceptual and put forward to encourage discussion. As with any complex plan of this sort, we realize that "the devil is in the details."

For specificity, following a general description of the program, we illustrate it using a hypothetical set of parameters. These are in no way to be considered a proposed set of conditions. In almost every instance, the appropriate numbers would require medical, economic, and policy analysis far beyond the scope of this book. However, we believe the specific examples help in clarifying the more general statements.

The Two-Part Program

Part One: The Private Option

The private option is a premium-support plan to provide individual freedom in choosing any approved health care plan subject to its availability and affordability. The objective of this option would be to maximize consumers' choices.

The Private Option Program.

When eligible, an individual would receive a premium-support subsidy for purchasing an insurance policy offered by private insurers on a nationwide insurance exchange.

Upon reaching eligibility, individuals having the same birth year would be assigned to a single cohort for that calendar year.

Only policies approved for the exchange would qualify for the subsidy. To be listed, a policy could not exclude coverage of pre-existing conditions or allow cancellation for new circumstances for individuals entering the program. Further, the policy conditions must be uniform for the entire cohort.

The support for a policy would be the lesser of (a) the policy cost or (b) a current maximum limit for the individual's cohort. (As an alternative, a more complex procedure could be included allowing means testing and health status in setting the maximum limits for individuals.)

In the base year (i.e., the first year of the overall private option) the maximum limit would be set relative to historical costs for Medicare. Following the base year, the maximum limit for each new cohort would be redefined in a manner analogous to wage-indexing in the Social Security program. That is, the initial-year maximum limit would be reset for the cohort in the light of health-care cost trends. The intent: each cohort starts on equal footing.

For each cohort, the maximum limit for subsequent years would be increased annually at the lesser of the general health care cost growth rate or a standard growth rate to be defined.

The first two years following eligibility would be a trial period. An individual could choose not to enroll until the end of the trial period or if enrolled would be free to change from one plan to another or to the public option without loss of coverage for pre-existing conditions.

Following the trial period, the individual would be free to change policies or to transfer to the public option with the stipulation that pre-existing conditions not covered by the individual's existing policy would not be protected in the new policy.

Part Two: The Public Option

The public option comprises three interlocking components: one, entitled "acute care," oriented to acute, preventive, restorative, and ameliorative care; a second, entitled "limited major medical," designed to pick up higher-cost chronic care and most major medical procedures; and a third, entitled "public major medical," as a final shield to protect from extremely high-cost, non-elective procedures. The objective of the public option would be to provide care in consonance with the concept of Healthy Normal Aging, which includes acknowledging that as age-related health care costs increase, the individual ought to assume a greater share of the economic burden.

The eligible age for the public option would be the same as for the private option and would cover pre-existing conditions. An individual choosing to enroll in the public option initially would be required to sign on to all three components, the acute care and public major medical components requiring no enrollment fees and a limited major medical policy to be purchased by the individual. After a specified number of years, continuation in limited major medical would become optional.

As with the private option, the first two years of the public option would be a trial period and following that period the individual would be free to change policies and options, subject to the proviso on pre-existing conditions.

Acute care: For this plan, there would not be an enrollment fee. Deductibles would be small or zero. Modest co-payment rates based on a patient's ability to pay would be assessed for care received. The postulate underlying co-paying is that, aside from periodic medical exams and counseling sessions, no medical service should be free to the beneficiary. Coverage of co-payments by ancillary insurance plans would be prohibited.

A broad range of medical services would be provided. Non-traditional medical practices could qualify for coverage when demonstrated to be effective. A single annual maximum expenditure limit would be applied for general care, including all aspects (hospital, MD, drugs, equipment, etc.). This amount would be defined relative to historical Medicare costs.

Higher co-payments would be assessed for proprietary drugs when suitable generic alternatives are available. No coverage would be permitted for commercially promoted proprietary prescription drugs.

Periodic review by a panel of representative medical professionals would define treatment categories that would be handled separately from general health care services. These would be elective high-cost, non-recurring or long-interval procedures or ongoing high-cost procedures judged to significantly improve the quality of life for the individual. These procedures would be exempt from the annual expenditure limit for general care. Specific formulas would be used to define out-of-pocket costs to the individual.

Limited major medical: This would be a private insurance supplement designed to cover high-cost chronic care and major-medical acute care up to an intermediate expenditure limit. That intermediate expenditure limit would be established relative to historical spending patterns. It would cover costs that exceed the maximum expenditure limit for general care under the specifications of acute care; it would not apply to the exempt categories described above.

At enrollment, individual purchase of a Limited Major Medical policy meeting or exceeding specified standards would be mandatory. This insurance supplement would be listed on the same nationwide exchange as the policies in the private option. The exchange would also list a publicly managed policy meeting the minimum standards. Each policy offered would have a single premium for the entire class of eligible individuals; there would be no age-dependent premiums.

For higher income individuals, payment for limited major medical would come primarily from the beneficiary. There would be low- and moderate-income premium support designed to cover all of the cost of the minimum standard policy for the lowest income individuals and that would retrogressively decline for higher income individuals.

The initial premium-support limit in the base year would be set in light of the actual experience with health care costs. Thereafter the maximum subsidy parameters would be indexed taking into account national economic growth. At a designated age, limited major medical would become optional.

Public major medical: The public major medical component as a last defense against extraordinarily high costs would take effect for expenditures above the limited major medical limits.

Public major medical would normally apply only to non-elective procedures and would specifically exclude certain procedures.

In cases where an individual has elected to discontinue limited major medical insurance, public major medical would not cover the gap. That gap would be the private responsibility of the individual.

Configurations

It is obvious that within the generalities stated above, one has great flexibility in designing a total program. We do not pretend that we have the wisdom and knowledge to say what the proper set of conditions and parameters ought to be. It all depends very much on what one hopes to accomplish. We believe that what those conditions and parameters ought to be is worth serious discussion.

One of Many Possible Examples

To better illustrate the nature of the program, in Table A we choose a partial set of conditions and parameters. What might our program look like if it had been set up to begin in 2008? The 2008 date for this hypothetical program is chosen to take advantage of data from KFF and Dartmouth. A hypothetical program as it would appear in 2008 is as follows.

Eligible Age for Both Private and Public Options: 65 years (and remains fixed)

Private Option

No means test or health status adjustments. The maximum is uniform for an entire age cohort.

In the base year, the maximum limit on the subsidy is set slightly higher than the median expenditure of the most cost-efficient quintile Hospital Health Referrals in 2007: $7,200 (Dartmouth).

In subsequent years, allow the maximum subsidy to increase at the same rate as U.S. per capita GDP.

Public Acute Care

No annual deductible.

Annual physical exams and counseling would be provided at no cost. Co-payment for other diagnostic office visits: $10.

Co-payments would range from 5% for individual incomes up to $10,000, increasing linearly to 10% for individual incomes of $50,000 or greater. A 20% co-payment surcharge applies to proprietary drugs for which medically appropriate generics are available.

General health care services would include the current Medicare array plus other annual services, including: insulin, hearing tests (and an allowance for hearing aids), eye examinations (and an allowance for eyeglasses), dental examinations (and an allowance for dental care), an allowance for physical therapy, an allowance for chiropractic services, and an allowance for acupuncture.

The maximum limit for total general health care expenditures in the base year: $14,000.

In subsequent years, the maximum limit would increase at the same rate as U.S. per capita GDP.

High-cost procedures, among others excluded from the acute care expenditure ceiling, include: knee and hip joint replacement, for which co-payments for these procedures could be amortized over a period of five years at zero interest, and chemo-therapy for rheumatoid arthritis, for which co-payments would be 5%.

Limited Major Medical

The minimum standard for insurance policies:

Insurance would be mandatory to age 80. Thereafter, optional.

Coverage for general health care in the base year would extend from $14,000–$75,000. The upper limit is chosen to cover the majority of end-of-life care cases (Dartmouth). Coverage would not apply to the exempt elective high-cost services specified in acute care.

In subsequent years, the limits on limited major medical coverage would increase at the rate of per capita GDP.

There would be a flat 10% co-payment.

Insurance policies in the base year would be subsidized at a declining rate from an estimated 100% of the minimum standard policy cost for individual incomes up to 150% of the federal poverty line (~$15,000) to 0% for incomes greater than $50,000.

Insurance subsidy limits would be indexed by per capita GDP growth.

Individuals would be permitted to purchase insurance policies exceeding the minimum standards (e.g., a lower co-payment rate, a higher maximum expenditure limit).

Public Major Medical

Payments entirely from public funds.

Except under unusual circumstances, elective procedures would not be covered.

Specific procedures to be excluded from coverage: all organ transplants, except kidney replacement.

Based on the hypothetical program, the following displays selected sample cases based on the hypothetical program for 2008. (> $20,000 per year) Public Option cases plus the 10% and 90% 2006 average-cost cases from KFF. In each case, it is assumed that three diagnostic visits at $150 each are made per year. Calculations are rounded to the nearest $10. An unsubstantiated guesstimate is made that a limited major medical policy meeting the minimum standard could be purchased on the exchange for $3,600 per year.

Public Option Case	Cost to Beneficiary (includes insurance premium)	Percent of Income	Cost to Private Insurance	Cost to Public System
Income: $10,000 End-of-life care: $80,000 (Cost absorbed by public)	($3,780)	(38%)	$57,950	$22,320
Income: $35,000 General health care: $6,000 Chemotherapy: $45,000	$5,080	14%	$35,150	$14,830
Income: $40,000 General health care: 5,000 Rheumatoid arthritis drugs: $20,000	$3,740	9%	$0	$25,310
Income: $50,000 General health care: $3,000 Hip replacement: $60,000 (amortize 5 yrs, 1st yr total public)	$5,130	10%	$0	$61,920
Income: $80,000 General health care: $6,000 Heart transplant: $100,000	$39,080	49%	$57,950	$13,020
Income: $10,000 Total health care: $3,910 (avg. 90% of 2006 cases, KFF)	$230	2%	$0	$7,730
Income: $10,000 Total health care: $48,210 (avg. 10% of 2006 cases, KFF)	$2,440	24%	$32,500	$17,320
Income: $50,000 Total health care: $3,910 (avg. 90% of 2006 cases, KFF)	$4,020	8%	$0	$3,940
Income: $50,000 Total health care: $48,210 (avg. 10% of 2006 cases, KFF)	$6,740	13%	$32,500	$13,020

Final Comments

First, the numbers that would apply to a realistic start date (e.g., 2020) would be much larger than those portrayed above. Second, it is obvious that a great deal of tinkering could and would be necessary to construct a program that hangs together. It would be important that the private and public options be truly competitive and that the cost burden be appropriately distributed between the income levels of all recipients. Third and most important, the feasibility of an approach of this sort is crucially dependent on how the private insurance market reacts. For example, a key question is how would the insurance industry price a uniform national pool for limited major medical and how would that compare with private option premiums?

References

Chapter 1

Thomas, Dylan. *Collected Poems*. 1953.

Berger, Thomas. *Little Big Man*. Boston, New York, London: Little, Brown and Company, 1989.

Burton, John and William Hall. *Taking Charge of Your Health*. Baltimore, Maryland: The Johns Hopkins University Press, 2010.

Holmes, Oliver Wendell. Quoted in the above cited reference [Burton].

Chapter 2 (no references)

Chapter 3

Monty Python and the Holy Grail. DVD. Columbia Tristar Home Entertainment, National Film Trustee Company, Ltd. Python (Monty) Pictures, Ltd., 1976.

Pilkington, Ed. "Pharmageddon: How America Got Hooked On Killer Prescription Drugs." *The Guardian*, 9 June 2011; http://www.guardian.co.uk/world/2011/jun/09/us-drugs-oxycodone-painkillers-florida?INTCMP=SRCH [accessed August 2012]

Chapter 4–5 (no references)

Chapter 6 and Appendix A

Hansen, R.W. and Robert Higgs (ed.). *Hazardous to Our Health? FDA Regulation of Health Care Products.* Oakland: The Independent Institute, 1995, 13–27.

———. Illustration A (the diagram was reprinted with permission from the publisher of the book, *Hazardous to Our Health? FDA Regulation of Health Care Products.* All rights reserved. © 1995, The Independent Institute, 100 Swan Way, Oakland, California 94621-1428; www.independent.org.

Boissel, J.P. "Impact of Randomized Clinical Trials on Medical Practices." *Controlled Clinical Trials.* Eds. Hasford, Knatterud, Fisher, and Messerer. New York: Elsevier Science Pub Co., 1989, 10:4 (Suppl 1) 120–134.

Bohenheimer, T. "Uneasy Alliances—Clinical Investigators and the Pharmaceutical Industry." *New Engl J Med* 2000, 342: 1539-44.

Sample, Ian. "Medical Ghostwriters Face Fraud Label." *The Guardian Weekly,* 12–18 August 2011, page 32.

Managed Care. http//www.ncbi.nlm.nih.gov. National Library of Medicine, 2011

Angell, M. "The Pharmaceutical Industry—To Whom Is It Accountable." *New Engl J Med* 2000, 1902–1904.

Chapter 7 (no references)

Chapter 8
Wikipedia. Search "Youth International Party," www.wikipedia.org [accessed 2011].

Wikipedia. Search "List of countries by life expectancy," wikipedia.org [accessed 2011].

Chapter 9

Wikipedia. Search "Switzerland Health Insurance," www.wikipedia. org (and from the author's personal insurance payments in Switzerland).

Canada Medical Health Plan, www.canadian-healthcare.org

Massachusetts State Health Reform, AARP.org/Massachusetts

California state health plan, www.healthcareforall.org

Alaska health information, www.healthcare.gov/alaskataskforce

Chapter 10

U.S. Department of Health and Human Services. The <u>Centers for Medicare & Medicaid Services (CMS)</u>. Medicare. http://www. medicare.gov coverage-basics, July 5, 2011.

Grisham, John. *The Rainmaker.* Arrow (Random House), 1996.

Chapter 11 and Appendix B

Federal Hospital Insurance and Federal Supplementary Medical Insurance Trust Funds. 2011 Annual Report of the Boards of Trustees.

Debt Reduction Task Force (Pete Domenici and Dr. Alice Rivlin, co-chairs). "Restoring America's Future." November 2010: Bipartisan Policy Center,

Domenici-Rivlin Task Force, President Obama, and Chairman Ryan. "Side-by-Side Comparison." April 22, 2011: Bipartisan Policy Center.

U.S. Congress. Congressional Budget Office. "Roadmap for America's Future." Letter to Honorable Paul Ryan, January 27, 2010.

_____. Letter to Honorable Ryan, November 17, 2010 (preliminary analysis of "A Longterm Plan for Medicare and Medicaid," Rivlin-Ryan).

_____. "Path to Prosperity." Letter to Honorable Ryan, April 5, 2011.

The Dartmouth Institute for Health Policy & Clinical Practice. "The Dartmouth Atlas of Health Care." www.dartmouthatlas.org (referred to as Dartmouth).

The Henry J. Kaiser Family Foundation. "Fast Facts." facts.kff.org (referred to as KFF).

_____. "Focus on Health Care Reform: Summary of the New Health Reform Law," April 15, 2011 (Patient Protection and Affordable Care Act).

Chapter 12

Stohler, Jacqueline. (Music photo and text.) Basel, Switzerland: Musiktherapie, Medizin/Onkologie, St. Clara Hospital, www.Jacqueline.Stohler@claraspital.ch.

Chapter13–14 (no references)

About the Authors

Thomas C. Jones, M.D.

Born in 1937 and raised in Medina, Ohio, he graduated from Allegheny College in Meadville, Pennsylvania, in 1958 and, to follow in his father's medical footsteps, he attended and graduated from Case Western Reserve Medical School in 1962. He served as an intern and completed his residency in medicine at Cornell University Medical College, The New York Hospital, from 1962 through 1967, including a one-year fellowship in infectious diseases.

He served as captain in the United States Air Force stationed at Clark Air Base in the Philippines from July 1967 to August 1969.

He did cell research at The Rockefeller University in New York, and completed an infectious diseases fellowship from 1969 to 1972.

He was assistant professor of medicine and public health, then associate professor of medicine and public health at Cornell University Medical College; then professor and chief of the division of international medicine, Department of Medicine, Cornell University Medical College, New York (1972–1985). He is emeritus adjunct professor of medicine and public health at Weill-Cornell Medical College, New York, to the present.

He was medical expert and then head of the division of infectious diseases, dermatology and asthma at Sandoz Pharmaceutical Ag., Basle, Switzerland (1985–1995).

He was head of Clinical Research Associates, Basle, Switzerland (1995–2005).

Jones wrote *The Medical Care of Refugees* (Oxford University Press, New York, 1987). He has published over 200 research articles in the medical literature. He was the first editor of the *Brazilian Journal of Infectious Diseases* (1996–2001).

His principal philosophy about health care is described in this book and includes the need for transparency in all aspects of health care, universal attention to basic needs of nutrition and health everywhere in the world, and a careful understanding of the need for quality of life care at the end of life, not heroic measures to extend life. As noted in this book, he also includes the requirement of each individual to fill their lives with humor, commitment to activity and pleasure, and to avoid all needless drugs or devices from even the most imposing sources.

I have added the following photograph to remind us all of two things: in addition to our need to stay mobile and healthy, part of our fun will always be interacting with youth—whether they be our children, grandchildren, nieces, nephews, or friends. If we do not get our government's finances and national health care in order, it is the young people who will have to pay for our mistakes.

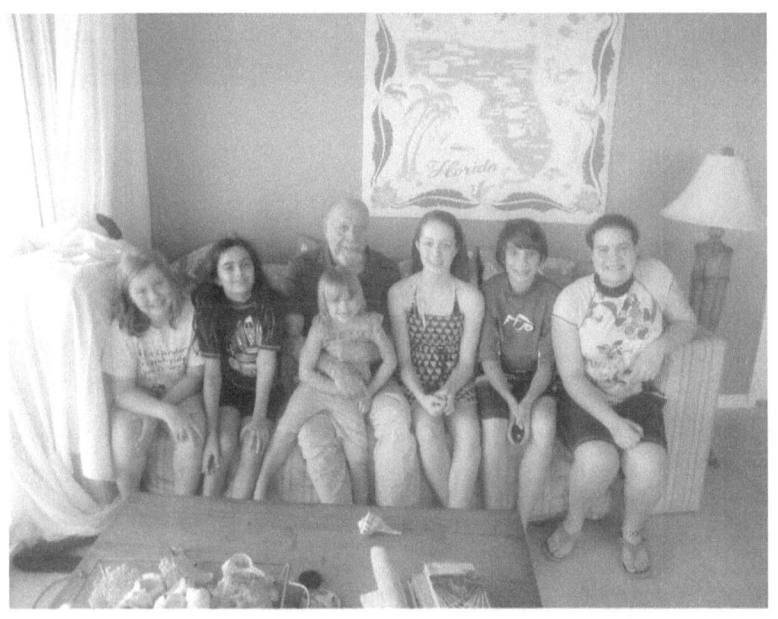

Figure 7. The author with his grandchildren in Florida.

This book was inspired by the book *Taking Charge of Your Health* by John Burton and William Hall. This author is indebted to the early participation of John and his wife, Lynda, in thinking about and editing this book. They provided important guidance at the outset but decided not to continue—probably for several reasons, among which it is likely that they disagree with my assessment of the impending health care crisis in the United States, and my assessment that primary health care providers are not in a proper position to make key decisions regarding their patients' health. The Burtons's opinions may be shared by many, but only time will make the final verdict. The author's son, Stefan, and his wife, Lauri, provided important information on the excellent health care system in Minnesota. The author's daughter, Phoebe, provided details of health care in Florida so that this book could be as specific as possible in guiding those in search of retirement options, assisted living, or nursing homes. Both my son's and daughter's observations also added much needed optimism concerning health care for elders in the United States.

John F. Cotton, M.S.

John was born in Meadville, Pennsylvania, in 1934, where he graduated from Meadville High School. In 1957, he graduated from Allegheny College with a major in physics (where he met Thomas C. Jones). He attended Princeton University Graduate School, September 1957–June 1959, followed by two years in the United States Army at Fort Riley, Maryland. He was program director for Undersea Warfare in Silver Spring, Maryland, April 1962–November 1965; assistant to the director, State and Local Finances Project, George Washington University, April 1966–August 1968; Vermont representative to the New England Regional Commission and deputy budget director and assistant to the governor, state of Illinois, May 1969–January 1973. He remained in Illinois, first as vice president and fellow at the Stevenson Institute, then director of Corporate Planning at Dekalb Ag. Research, April 1974–November 1977.

In November 1977, he moved to California. He was vice president for corporate development at Dynapol in Palo Alto, California, then a trustee for Liquidation until April 1981. In June 1984, he became a student at California State Polytechnic University (Cal Poly), Pomona, where he received a master's degree in architectural engineering in May 1989. He was a lecturer at Cal Poly and a manager of architectural computing at the University of California at Berkeley, then associate professor of architecture at Cal Poly, June 1989–August 2000.

He is active and in good health.

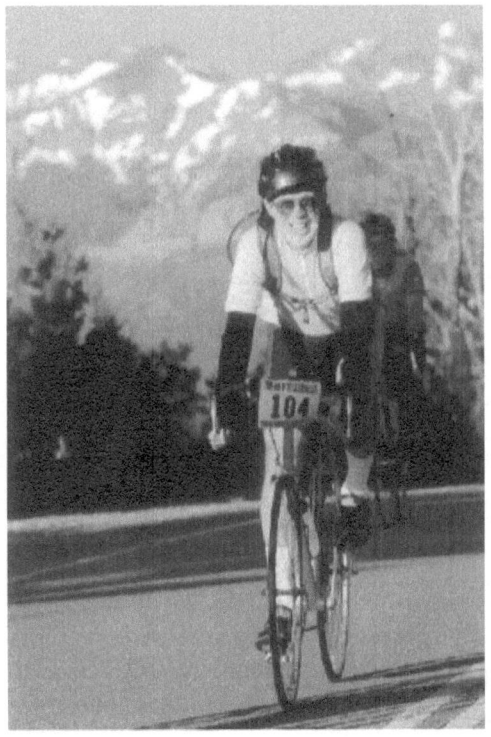

Figure 8. John Cotton at 70 years old in the High Sierras.

At retirement, John chose not to enroll in the CalPers supplement to medicare program. He has retained the same PPO insurance he held while a faculty member at Cal Poly SLO. To the disapproval of Thomas C. Jones, John's position toward health care is drawn from his philosophy of care for an old automobile he once owned—an adult toy, and for his bike: If it ain't broke, don't fix it. There are always strange new quirks so, be sure it's broke before you try to fix it. And sometimes, you just don't fix it.

Betsy M. Chalfin, M.Ed.

Betsy graduated with a B.A. in history from Northwestern University, Evanston, Illinois, and received a master's degree in special education from the University of Illinois, Chicago, in 1977. On returning to New York, she happened upon a temporary job in the new division of international medicine at Cornell University Medical College and decided she preferred the challenges of medical administration to teaching. She was program coordinator for the division of international medicine from 1978–1984, where she administered a number of international programs, including the Cornell Thailand Project that provided medical care to displaced Cambodians in Khao I Dang Refugee Camp (1979–1983). She went on to serve as the medical program director for the International Rescue Committee, New York, in 1984 and 1985. She was copyeditor of *Medical Care of Refugees*, by Thomas C. Jones and Richard Sandler (Oxford University Press, New York, 1987) and research assistant to the well-known author Marilyn French. In 1991, she became director of residency for recruitment and the academic administrator in the Department of Neurology at the Mount Sinai School of Medicine, New York; in 1998 she became administrator for the Department of Neurology under Susan B. Bressman, M.D., at the Beth Israel Medical Center, New York. She was copyeditor for the *Brazilian Journal of Infectious Diseases* 1996–2001. Now she spends her energy on gardening and rehabbing historic houses.

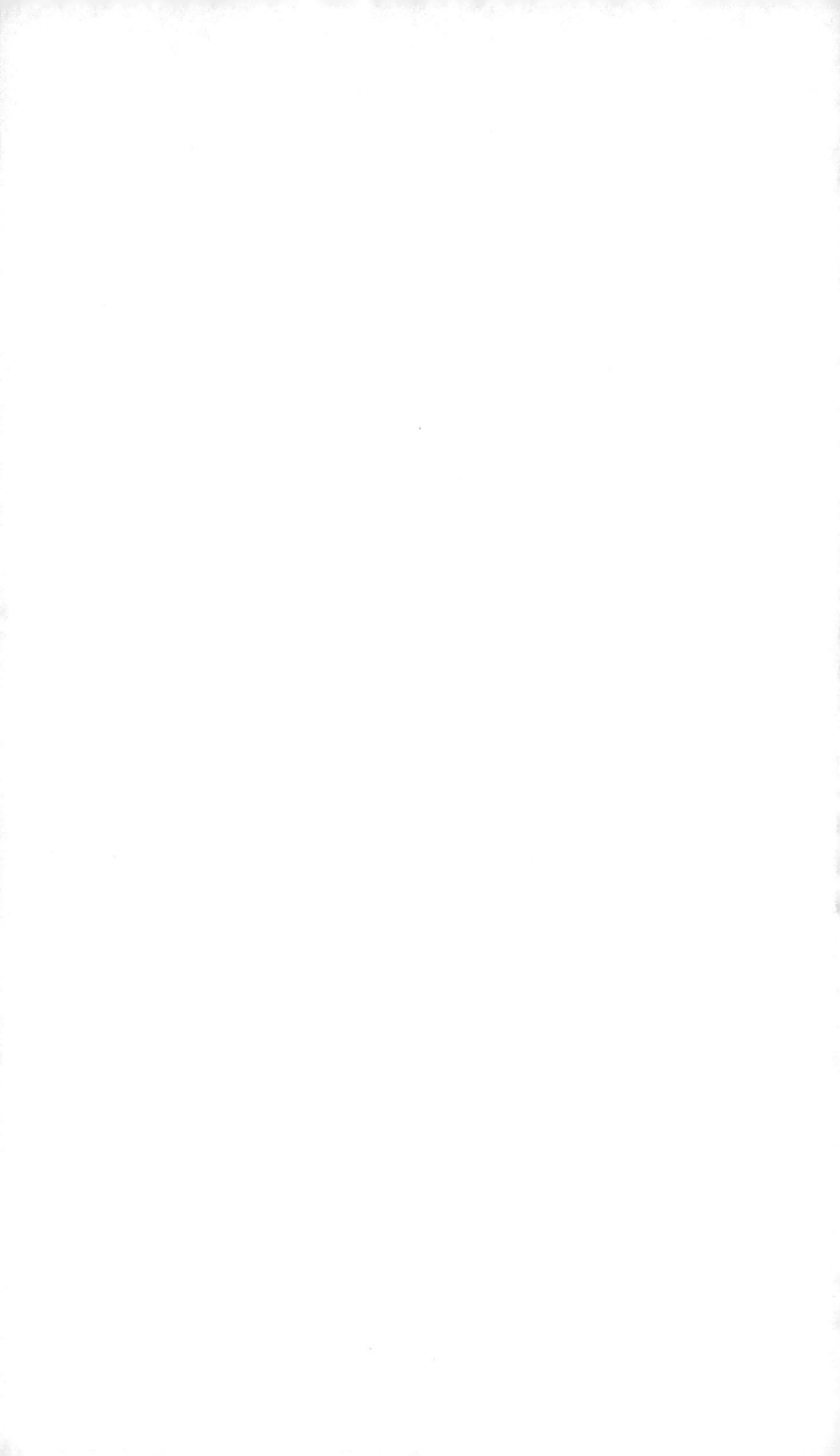